ATOPIC DERMATITIS

ATOPIC DERMATITIS

Satish Udare MD DVD
Professor
Department of Dermatology
MGM Medical College
Navi Mumbai, Maharashtra, India

Foreword
Hemangi Jerajani

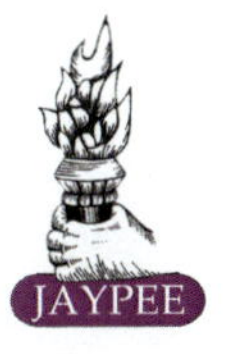

The Health Sciences Publisher
New Delhi | London | Panama

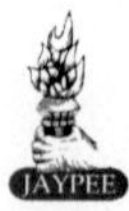 **Jaypee Brothers Medical Publishers (P) Ltd**

Headquarters

Jaypee Brothers Medical Publishers (P) Ltd
4838/24, Ansari Road, Daryaganj
New Delhi 110 002, India
Phone: +91-11-43574357
Fax: +91-11-43574314
Email: jaypee@jaypeebrothers.com

Overseas Offices

J.P. Medical Ltd
83 Victoria Street, London
SW1H 0HW (UK)
Phone: +44 20 3170 8910
Fax: +44 (0)20 3008 6180
Email: info@jpmedpub.com

Jaypee-Highlights Medical Publishers Inc
City of Knowledge, Bld. 235, 2nd Floor, Clayton
Panama City, Panama
Phone: +1 507-301-0496
Fax: +1 507-301-0499
Email: cservice@jphmedical.com

Jaypee Brothers Medical Publishers (P) Ltd
17/1-B Babar Road, Block-B, Shyamoli
Mohammadpur, Dhaka-1207
Bangladesh
Mobile: +08801912003485
Email: jaypeedhaka@gmail.com

Jaypee Brothers Medical Publishers (P) Ltd
Bhotahity, Kathmandu
Nepal
Phone: +977-9741283608
Email: kathmandu@jaypeebrothers.com

Website: www.jaypeebrothers.com
Website: www.jaypeedigital.com

Atopic Dermatitis

First Edition: 2019

ISBN: 978-93-5270-227-5

Printed at: Samrat Offset Pvt. Ltd.

Dedicated to

My team at 'Disha' and 'Sparkle' Skin and Aesthetic Centres and my Team at MGM Medical College

Contributors

Pranjal Ahire MBBS, DNB
Lecturer
MGM Medical College
Navi Mumbai, Maharashtra India

Satish Udare MD DVD
Professor
MGM Medical College
Navi Mumbai, Maharashtra, India

Saurabh Jindal MD, DNB
Former Associate Professor
MGM Medical College
Navi Mumbai, Maharashtra India

Shaurya Rohatgi MD
Former Associate Professor
MGM Medical College
Navi Mumbai, Maharashtra India

Shylaja Somshwar MBBS, DBD, DNB
Associate Professor
MGM Medical College
Navi Mumbai, Maharashtra India

Foreword

I am delighted to write this foreword for the compilation of chapters written by my own colleagues from MGM Medical College, Kamothe, Navi Mumbai, Maharastra, India, on atopic dermatitis.

Dr Satish Udare, Professor in the Department of Dermatology deserves accolades for the entire project, from conception to actual achievement, single headedly. He has managed to bring all the diverse authors with theirs distinctive style efficiently together in unique endeavor. Atopic dermatitis is a complex disease with a large spectrum of clinical features in various ages. The Indian subcontinent experience is unique and differs from the Western counter part due to socio-geological reasons. Dr Udare has made this print very succinctly in each and every chapter.

The first chapter in the book is written by Dr Satish Udare to give us the glimpses of historical personalities and journey of atopic dermatitis. Dr Saurabh Jindal, the then Associate Professor of Dermatology, has meticulously discussed the pathogenesis of atopic dermatitis with interplay of CD4/CD8 cells, the roll of IL-2, IL-10 and other inflammatory mediators.

The varied clinical features, especially found more commonly in this part of word is compiled in a simple style by Dr Pranjal Salunke, Assistant Professor of Dermatology. Dr Shylaja Someshwer has done a herculean task of compiling all the classifications and the diagnosis in a readable style. Dr Shaurya Rohatgi, Assistant Professor deserves a pat on his shoulder for writing the chapter on management of atopic dermatitis. He has included all the medical therapy with new and old for comparison.

For an all-rounder clinician, it is important to know about the prevailing thought of alternative therapies. Dr Udare has done exclusive work in this field, and therefore it is apt that he has written the chapter on complementary medicines.

Overall, it is a book written on atopic dermatitis by my colleagues in a very easy and likeable style. They have definitely succeeded in bringing out the best talents within themselves.

I am sure the general practitioners, students and clinicians will find this book very user friendly and handy.

Happy reading to all of you.

Hemangi Jerajani
Professor and HOD
Department of Dermatology
MGM Hospital,
Kamothe, Navi Mumbai, Maharashtra, India

Preface

When I was studying dermatology the incidence of 'Atopic dermatitis' in our Indian population and especially in general hospitals in Mumbai was minimal. As I started my practice I started noticing few cases. For me it was almost like a new entity to be diagnosed. I distinctly remember when first time Mometasone was launched and was indicated in children with atopic dermatitis, one of the senior professors got up and declared that 'we may not need it as there is no such entity as atopic dermatitis in India'. I stood up and said that it is present definitely, more so in children from NRI parents, I was ridiculed. But soon everybody had realized that the incidence is on the rise, probably as we are becoming 'Developing country'.

I was chief coordinator of a small conference on atopic dermatitis when I really got interested in subject, as the depth of my knowledge about the disease increased. As I continued to see more patients, their sufferings, their parents' plight, I thought I should make everybody aware that this condition is there, is increasing and becoming a menace, hence proper knowledge of the condition and its management should be understood and learned by all.

I hope my efforts in this direction are helpful to all and will result in better management of the sufferers.

I am thankful to my team of contributors who have done excellent job in the same direction. I am thankful to Shri Jitendar P Vij (Group Chairman), Mr Ankit Vij (Group President), Ms Ritu Sharma (Director—Content Strategy), Ms Chetna Malhotra Vohra (Associate Director—Content Strategy), Ms Sunita Katla (PA to Group Chairman and Publishing Manager) of M/s Jaypee Brothers Medical Publishers (P) Ltd, New Delhi, for helping me in completing my endeavor.

Satish Udare

Contents

History and Epidemiology

Satish Udare

INTRODUCTION

Atopic dermatitis (AD) is a disease characterized by itching, by acute exacerbations and remissions. The disease starts right from early infancy and in many cases continues till adulthood disturbing not only the individual but entire family.

Atopic dermatitis is chronic relapsing disease and has characteristic patterns according to age and has varied presentation. It has association with both genetic factors and environmental influences and has association with other diseases like asthma, hay fever, allergic rhinitis which together form so called "atopic diathesis". Though lot of research has been done till date, the disease still is an enigma and presently on rise world over, more so in India.

HISTORY[1]

In the earlier days during late 18th century there was confusion about the disease, the fight was from word eczema to dermatitis, whether it is a AD or atopiform eczema, is it an intrinsic or extrinsic eczema, etc., and till date, there is conflicting evidences about atopy and AD associations. The disease has been given various names by various people with different perspectives, as observed by its different manifestations almost like blind men and elephant. These different manifestations were described under many different headings, such as prurigo, eczemas, and lichens. Many descriptive terms were used to describe different types of eruptions and variants of AD, such as prurigo of Hebra, Besnier's prurigo, popular urticaria and lichen circumscriptum, etc. Vidal described lichen simples, Broq described as neurodermatitis localized or generalized forms, many years it was described as prurigo of Besnier. By early nineteenth century many famous dermatologists described this chronic itchy dermatosis by various different names, Erasmus Williums first time described infantile eczema group. But gradually precursor picture of atopic eczema was clearly emerging. In 1923 Coca and Cooke with help of Perry proposed the name atopy—meaning" strange disease" in ancient greek language or "not in right place" or "strange" to designate a type of heritable hypersensitivity to common environmental allergens noted in asthma and hay fever[2] on classification of the phenomena of hypersensitiveness. Besnier earlier had described the diathesis of atopy with asthma, hay fever, allergic rhinitis and gastrointestinal allergies.

Hill and Sulzberger described the natural history and clinical symptoms of AD from infancy to adulthood.[3] Wise and Shulzberger suggested term dermatitis than eczema, Ackerman wanted to expunge word eczema.[4] Various others chipped in knowledge pieces, such as use of patch test by Jadasohn, role of allergy, transferable hypersensitivity, histamine, house dust mite, etc. Role of t1 and t2 immunity response was elucidated later as disease was recognized. The diagnostic criteria started emerging and Hanifan and Rajka[5] came forward with the criteria for diagnosis of AD and since then there were many modifications. Still controversies exists about inside out and outside in theories, atopiform dermatitis and others.[6]

First documented atopic individual was most likely emperor Octavianus Augustus, who suffered from extremely itchy skin, seasonal rhinitis and tightness of the chest (probably Bible mentions about AD when it says "in the beginning, there was the itch).

In India, there are no clear cut evidence of atopic-like dermatitis from ancient literature but the disease is noticed and reported increasingly now.

Considering the different theories or lack of knowledge of exact etiology of disease, it is obvious that the therapy part also kept on modifying. There were messy external therapies in past and toxic chemicals internally, such as arsenic and mercury. Bloodletting, emetics and laxatives aimed at correcting diathesis and clearing the internal abnormalities. Lassar paste and tars were used initially, cortisone was introduced by 1950s[7] which were miraculous, antibiotics were added as the theory of superantigen was introduced, lastly newer treatments with calcineurin inhibitors and biologics were added recently.

EPIDEMIOLOGY

Epidemiology, (term epi means upon, demos means people and logos means study, the word is derived from greek language).[8] is study of what is present upon population, its distribution amongst population and factors responsible for it. Incidence means new cases and prevalence means number of actual cases. The study usually will identify risk and environmental factors so as to prevent the disease and suggest therapeutic approaches.

The exact incidence is difficult to assert because of varied diagnostic criteria and prevalence of disease may vary in different regions of the same country. As AD has both genetic background and environmental influences the incidence varies greatly over the world, age, climatic and socioeconomic conditions.[9]

Prevalence of AD in preschool children in United Kingdom is 21.0%, meanwhile in China it is only 3.07%. Overall it was observed that prevalence is increasing where it was lower and leveling where it was high.[10] International study of asthma and allergies in childhood, (which undertook 12 months study of prevalence of symptoms of asthma, allergic rhinoconjunctivitis and atopic eczema) was established in 1991 and collected data in 3 phases on questionnaire-based study in more than 100 countries[11] (issac, phase 1).

Incidence in various countries had been found to vary between 3 and 20.5%[11] [more than 37,000 children]. From India, 14 different centers were studied. All centers except Kottayam (Kerala) reported a 12-month period prevalence between 2.4% and 6% while Kottayam reported a prevalence of >9%.[12]

In Isaac, phase 3, prevalence of atopic diseases in more than a million children from around 100 countries has been determined by standard questionnaire-based survey.

Current eczema was defined as the presence of flexural rash in preceding 12 months, while severe disease was defined as one or more nights with disturbed sleep per week. Comparison of data between Isaac phase 1 and 3 has confirmed that worldwide prevalence of AD is rising, especially in younger children.[12] As far as prevalence of AD is concerned in the studied age groups, i.e. 6–7 years and 13–14 years, most of the centers participating showed rising incidence. So was the scenario with prevalence of severe atopic eczema in population-based studies on epidemiology of AD in India. In India, the disease was rare initially but now has fairly common occurrence and it is apparently on rise as it is becoming a developing country. The data is not rampant in Indian literature, though whatever data available suggests that the clinical manifestations and course and severity may not be same as Western literature depicts (prevalence is some of the Indian studies ranges from 0.42–0.38).[13,14] They also reported onset age 2.5 years with 1.3:1 m:f ratio with type of disease depending on area involved, verity according to Scorad.

In India, the whole spectrum may still vary as we have cold and dry climate in north, west coastal warm humid and extremes of temperatures throughout the year. Winter exacerbations showing acute lesions in many areas, 40% gave history of atopy in family and 54% had history of atopy in self.

Lesion as acute type were more common in infants and chronic in later ages. Most epidemiological data that is available is based on hospital-based studies thus, not necessarily meant to determine the epidemiological trend.

A rising trend in AD has been observed in India also in last four decades.[15] A study from Bihar reported an incidence of 0.38% of the total number of outpatient attendees.[16]

Relatively recent hospital-based studies have also determined a low prevalence both in the northern and eastern part of the country. The reported prevalence among dermatology outpatient department attendees being 0.42% and 0.55%, respectively.[17,18] However, AD was the commonest dermatosis in children registered to a pediatric dermatology clinic where it constituted 28.46% of all registered patients. In contrast, only 0.01% (3 out of 2100) children in a south Indian study had AD. This relative rarity has been attributed to different dietary habits and climate.[19] These facts have been reflected in a hospital-based study where patients from urban areas outnumbered those from rural areas (1:0.3 for patients up to 1 year of age and 1:0.46 for patients beyond 1 year) and (1.8:1 for infants and 2.12:1 for children). Majority of the patients in the study by Sarkar and Kanwar belonged to middle class families (53.8% for up to 1 year and 57.57% afterwards) while minority of the patients was from poor strata (15.5% and 23.23%, respectively). Limitation of this data is that the stratification of the baseline population where the patients belonged considering area of residence and socioeconomic.

Status were not considered while majority of the patients in one study had aggravation of their eczema in the winters (62%) as a result of decreased moisture in the climate, 17% had aggravation in the summers, probably due to hyperhidrosis, itch and secondary skin infection. Similar was the findings of Dhar and Kanwar: Where 67.14% of infants had aggravation.

During winters prevalence of AD is variable from place to place as the environment plays a major role in its etiopathogenesis. AD is less severe in India than in western countries. Blood group O was found significantly less commonly in patients than in controls. How should ABO blood group be related somehow to AD was not discussed.

A lot is to be known in the Indian scenario on diagnostic criteria chosen but on the whole skin condition that often begins in infancy or early childhood, with 85–90% of cases appearing in the first 5 years of life. 45% by age of 6 months and around. Out of these 40% may resolve by age of 7–8 and around 60% by adulthood. The disease predominantly is of childhood, but it can also occur in adulthood for the first time. The disease usually resolve by puberty in 50% of patients, there is no difference in male or female distribution including the severity. The disease is present worldwide though incidence is more in developed countries and is on rise in developing countries. It is observed that it is more common in urban population than rural and also more prevalent in affluent classes, though it may be because of higher reporting and also according to hygiene hypothesis.[20]

The disease risk appears to be reduced in children in larger families.[21] The infections, exposure to environmental allergens, infants, washing, pollution, tobacco self or maternal, gut microflora, early feeding or longer breast feeding, live and inactivated vaccinations all have controversial role in developing AD. The disease has more incidence in families with history of atopic diathesis and in twin studies.

As depicted earlier it was long known about the association of several diseases, such as bronchial asthma, hay fever, allergic rhinitis, allergic conjunctivitis, gastrointestinal symptoms and other allergic manifestations, several family studies, twin studies has posively ascertained the association. It is observed in some individuals that as the skin lesions appear, the asthma tends to reduce and when asthma worsens the skin improves. Though in some individuals both may improve or worsen simultaneously.

NATURAL HISTORY OF THE DISEASE

This means once the disease has occurred in an individual how long it will last, when it might disappear and if and when it becomes severe. In various studies it was observed that upto 60% may resolve by 6 years, usually starts by 2 years in 60% of cases. 40% have intermittent disease and 10% may persists in adulthood.[22,24]

Patients with AD may develop "atopic march "in 30% people, may develop asthma, 66% may develop allergic sensitization, that is they develop food allergy, rhinitis.[23] Children with severe disease, more barrier damage and IgE aeroallergens are likely to develop atopic march.

The disease causes severe burden on families and society at large, children may miss school, affecting the scholastic performance, the emotional and behavioral changes lead to social isolations and psychological consequences ultimately leading to poor quality of life (this will be dealt in separately later). Working hours of parents, and adult patients and partners are severely affected leading to increased financial burden and adding to this is the cost of drugs and therapies.

Nutrition of the patients is routinely affected by drugs, allergies and disease severity.

REFERENCES

1. Taïeb A, Wallach D, Tilles G. The History of Atopic Eczema/ Dermatitis. In: Ring J, Przybilla B, Ruzicka T (Eds). Handbook of Atopic Eczema: Springer Berlin Heidelberg; 2006. p. 10-20.
2. Coca AF, Cooke RA. On classification of the phenomena of hypersensitiveness. J Immunol. 1923;6:63.
3. Mier PD. Earliest description of the atopic syndrome? Br J Dermatol. 1975;92:359.
4. Ackerman AB, Ragaz A. A Plea to expunge the word "eczema" from the lexicon of dermatology and dermatopathology. Arch Dermatol Res. 1982;272(3):407-20.
5. Hanifin J, Rajka G. Diagnostic features of atopic dermatitis. Acta Derm Venereol (Stockh) 1980;Supp. 92:44–7.
6. Bos JD. Atopiform dermatitis. BJD. 2002;147:426-9.
7. Debr´e R, et al. Cortisone therapy of eczema in infants. Arch Fr Pediatr. 1951;8:760-2.
8. Wikipedia.
9. Odhiambo JA, Williams HC, clayton TO, Robertoson CF, Asher MI; ISAAC phase. Three study Group. Global variations in prevalence of eczema symptons in children from ISAAC Phase Three. J Allergy clin Immunole. 2009;124(6):1251-8.
10. Williams, et al. Is eczema really on the increase worldwide? J Allergy clin Immunol. 2008;12(4): 947-54.
11. Asher mieur resp j 1995; 8, lancet 2006;368 (ISSAC, phase 1).
12. Worldwide variation in prevalence of symptoms of asthma, allergic rhinoconjuctivitis and atopic eczema: ISAAC. The International Study of Asthma and Alergies in Childhood (ISAAC) Steering committee. Lancet 1998;351(911):1225-32.
13. Dhar kanwar 1998 ped derm, sinha Indian j dermatol Venereol leprol 1972;38.
14. Kanwar AJ, Dhar S, Kaur S. Evaluation of minor clinical features of atopic dermatitis. Pediatr Dermatol. 1991;8:114-6.
15. Dhar S. Atopic dermatitis: Indian scenario. Indian J Dermatol Venereol Leprol. 1999;65:253-7.
16. Sinha PK. Clinical profile of infantile atopic eczema in Bihar. Indian J Dermatol Venereol Leprol. 1972:38:179-84.
17. Dhar S, Kanwar AJ. Epidemiology and clinical pattern of atopic dermatitis in north Indian pediatric population. Pediatr Dermatol. 1998;15:347-51.
18. Dhar S, Mandal B, Ghosh A. Epidemiology and clinical pattern of atopic dermatitis in 100 children seen in city hospital. Indian J Dermatol. 2002;47:202.
19. Karthikeyan K, Thappa DM, Jeevankumar B. Pattern of pediatric dermatoses in a referral center in south India. Indian Pediatr. 2004;41:373-7.
20. Karmaus W, Botezan C. Does higher number of siblings protect against the development of allergy and asthma? A review. J Epidemiol community Health. 2002;56:209-17.

21. Strachan DP. Family size, infection and Atopy: The first decade of the "hygiene hypothesis." Thorax. 2000;55 [Suppl 1]:S2–S10.
22. Ricci G, Patrizi A, Baldi E, Menna G, Tabanelli M, Masi M. Long-term follow-up of atopic dermatitis: retrospective analysis of related risk factors and association with concomitant allergic diseases. J Am Acad Dermatol. 2006 Nov;55(5):765-71.
23. van der Hulst AE, Klip H, Brand PL. Risk of developing asthma in young children with atopic eczema: a systemic reviews. J Allergy Clin Imunol. 2007;120(3):565-9.
24. Illi S1, von Mutius E, Lau S, Nickel R, Grüber C, Niggemann B, Wahn U; Multicenter Allergy Study Group. The natural course of atopic dermatitis from birth to age 7 years and the association with asthma. J Allergy Clin Immunol. 2004 May;113(5):925-31.

Etiology and Pathogenesis

Saurabh Jindal

INTRODUCTION

Atopic dermatitis (AD) is a chronic recurrent inflammatory disease. Incidence of AD is on the rise all over the world and this fact has been specially noted in urban population. AD erupts due to a complex interplay between genetic susceptibility genes, environmental and innate immunological factors ultimately leading to barrier damage. This barrier dysfunction plays a major role in the pathogenesis of AD leading to entry of allergens and microbes. Studies of asthma and atopy have shown that in etiology, the proportion of contributory factors is likely to be about 50% environment and 50% genes.[1]

GENETIC INFLUENCE

Genetic influence in AD is well known. This is supported by studies of twins. In two early genetic epidemiologic studies in population-based twin samples, the pairwise concordance rate was 0.72–0.86 for monozygotic twins and 0.21–0.23 for dizygotic twins.[2,3] In children with AD, it is particularly associated with the prevalence of atopic disease in their parent (maternal> paternal). Approximately 27% of children whose parents are not atopic develop AD versus 38% and 50%, respectively, of children with one or two affected parents.[4] Kaufman et al. reported that 58% of children developing allergic symptoms if one parent has allergies and 79% if both parents are affected.[5] A parental history of atopic respiratory disease increases the risk significantly more for IgE-associated than non-IgE associated AD. Significantly, eczema and allergic disease are associated with several single-gene Mendelian disorders, including Job's syndrome,[6,7] Netherton's syndrome,[8] thymic hypoplasia (Di George syndrome), cellular deficiency with immunoglobulins (Nezelof's syndrome), selective IgA deficiency, and Wiskott-Aldrich syndrome. AD candidate susceptibility genes have been identified the loci of which are illustrated in the table below (Table 2.1).

Surprisingly, many loci associated with AD overlap with known psoriasis loci (1q, 3q, 17q and 20p),[9] which is

Table 2.1: Candidates for susceptibility genes

1q21[9]

3p24–22[10]

3q21[11]

17q25[9]

3p26–24[12]

3q14[10]

4p15–14[12]

13q14[10]

15q14–15[10]

17q21[10]

18q11–12[12]

18q21[10]

20p[9]

unexpected because the two conditions are almost mutually exclusive in clinical practice. This shared locus overlies the epidermal differentiation complex (EDC). EDC is a cluster of genes encoding proteins found in the uppermost layers of the epidermis, which are of great importance for keratinocyte differentiation and skin-barrier maintenance.[13] Genes located in the EDC include loricrin (LOR), involucrin (IVL), filaggrin (FLG), the small proline-rich protein (SPRR) genes and the late cornified envelope (LCE) genes. Abnormal epidermal barrier function is consistently found in AD; and it is not clear whether the dry skin is only a consequence of the underlying immune inflammatory process or a cause of the inflammatory cascade.

Mutations found in FLG (loss-of-function mutations) suggest skin barrier deficiency as a major abnormality in AD.[14-16] FLG (filaggrin) appears to be the most important gene because more than 35 mutations in FLG are known to be associated with AD. Inheriting one null FLG mutation slightly increases one's risk of developing AD, and inheriting two mutations (either as a homozygote or a compound heterozygote) significantly increases one's risk. Between 42% and 79% of persons with one or more FLG null mutations will develop AD. The explanation for this is that FLG (expressed in the upper epidermis) has an important role in the aggregation of keratin filaments, which is necessary for the formation of the stratum corneum (SC).[17] Subsequently, within the SC, FLG is degraded to form a group of amino acids, collectively called the natural moisturizing factor (NMF). NMF plays a vital role in hydrating the SC. The same FLG mutation is also seen in ichthyosis vulgaris which is often seen in association with AD. FLG mutations have a very significant effect on the course of the atopic disease. They are more associated with AD that presents early in life, tends to persist into childhood and adulthood, and is associated with wheezing in infancy and asthma. FLG mutations are also associated with allergic rhinitis and keratosis pilaris, independent of AD. Hyperlinear palms are strongly associated with FLG mutations (71% positive predictive value). However, FLG mutations have also been seen in normal individuals who are unaffected (40% of carriers with FLG null mutations never have AD). As the FLG gene is located in or near psoriasis susceptibility (PSORS) 4 locus, FLG mutations were also studied in psoriasis patients, however no associations were found. Also, not all cases of AD are associated with FLG mutations and AD patients often demonstrate clinical findings consistent with a T-helper 2 (Th2) phenotype. Mutations in genes expressed by Th2 cells, especially the interleukin (IL)-4 gene promoter region, have been identified in patients with AD. A gene at 16p11.2–12 encoding the α chain of the IL-4 receptor has been linked to atopy.[18-20] A gain-of-function mutation in this α chain of the IL-4 has been associated with AD. Interestingly, overexpression of Th2 cytokines downregulates FLG protein expression in patients with AD. This could lead to an "acquired" FLG deficiency, resulting in or exacerbating AD. A polymorphism in the gene encoding the β-chain of the high affinity IgE receptor FCϵR1β has demonstrated a highly significant association with AD.[21] Variants in the RANTES gene promoter region have also been reported.[22] Another genetic influence contributing to abnormal barrier function is SPINK5 which encodes LEKTI, a serine protease inhibitor expressed at epithelial and mucosal surfaces. Although mutations in this gene determine Netherton's syndrome, variants in the gene have also been associated with AD.[23-25] LEKTI inhibits 2 serine proteases involved in inflammation and desquamation. Due to LEKTI underexpression, there is increase in serine proteases contributing to atopic inflammation and barrier dysfunction.

MATERNAL FACTORS

It has been observed that atopic disorders are more frequently transmitted to the child by mothers than by fathers.[26,27] Possible mechanisms are:
- Suppression of paternal genomic effects
- Intrauterine programming (a major factor of which is the balance between fetal nutrition and growth rate)
- Immunological sensitization through intrauterine exposure to food and environmental allergens which the mother is subjected to.

ENVIRONMENTAL FACTORS

Second to genetic factors, environmental factors seem to be the most likely modulating influences. In this context "hygiene hypothesis" has been proposed. According to this hypothesis, over-hygienic upbringing predisposes the child to AD through lessened exposure to environmental microbes. This could be due to the fact that early life microbial exposure contributes to immune system maturation so that atopic immune dysregulation associated with production of IgE antibody does not occur.[28] Early further evidence was provided when it was documented that exposure to hepatitis A virus, *Helicobacter pylori* or *Toxoplasma gondii* reduced the risk of atopy by more than 60%.[29] In contrast, it seems that exposure to respiratory pathogens is not associated with this effect.[29] The significant differences between rural and urban areas could also be explained by the increased levels of exposure to microbes in rural settings.

IMMUNE DYSREGULATION

The histologic feature of AD is the same as any eczematous disease, comprising of epidermal proliferation, lymphocytic infiltration of predominantly CD4+T cells into the dermis (and sometimes epidermis), and increased numbers of dermal macrophages and eosinophils.[30] A variety of functional abnormalities have been noted in these infiltrating cells as well as in circulating leukocytes.[31]

Biphasic Pattern of Cytokine Expression in Atopic Skin Lesions

The pattern of local cytokine expression plays an important role in modulating tissue inflammation, and in AD this pattern depends on the acuity or duration of the skin lesion. The expression of IL-4, IL-5, IL-13, and IFN-γ in skin biopsy specimens from clinically normal (uninvolved), acute (erythematous AD lesions of <3 days' duration), and chronic (>2 weeks' duration) skin lesions of patients with AD has been investigated by means of in situ hybridization.[32,33] Acute skin lesions are rich in TH-2 (IL-4 and IL-13) cytokine expression while chronic skin lesions show a switch to TH-1 pattern with an increased expression of IL-5 and IFN-γ and IL-12, with significant decrease in IL-4 and IL-13. IL-12 plays a key role in TH1-cell development, and its expression in eosinophils and/or macrophages is thought to initiate the switch to TH1-cell development in chronic skin lesions. These observations have led to the proposal that initiation of AD is driven by allergen-induced activation of TH2-type cells, whereas the chronic inflammatory response is dominated by a TH1-type response driven by the infiltration of IL-12-expressing eosinophils and macrophages, which accompanies the initial TH2 response.

Skin Directed Th2-like Cell response in AD

In 80% of children with AD, allergic rhinitis or asthma eventually develops. Many of these patients outgrow their AD as they are developing respiratory allergy. The explanation for this phenomenon is as follows: A patient may have allergic disease but its clinical expression is determined by local tissue allergen sensitization. There is also compartmentalization of the immune response in the skin or the respiratory mucosa. Thus, allergic diseases involve organ-specific allergic inflammatory responses and the mechanisms that control recruitment of TH2 lymphocytes to these different tissue sites determine the end clinical site of affection. If cutaneous leukocyte antigen (CLA) levels are measured in T cells, they are higher in the skin where allergen-induced reactions are taking place compared to the T cells isolated from the airways of patients with asthma.[34]

IgE-mediated Allergic Reactivity

Most persons with AD have a personal or family history of allergic rhinitis or asthma. 80% patients with AD have increased serum IgE antibodies against airborne or ingested protein antigens while 20% of patients with AD have normal serum IgE and no allergen reactivity[35,36] and the disease also occurs in agammaglobulinemic children with no IgE.[37] Thus, the role of IgE in this eczematous cutaneous disease remains tenuous and speculative and further research is needed in this area.

Cellular Immune Abnormalities

The exact role of cellular immune responses was speculated right from the days of noted dermatologist Kaposi. He was aware of some immune incompetence in patients with AD because of their susceptibility to widespread herpes simplex infections.[38] Later on other observers also noted reduced sensitivity of patients with AD to poison ivy and dinitrochlorobenzene (DNCB).[39] Immunohistochemical similarities of AD to contact allergy raised a paradox. Lesions that appear to reflect a cell-mediated immunological response actually are occurring in skin with reduced cellular immune responses.[40] This paradox could be due to Th1/Th2 immunologic dichotomy. The lesional studies have shown that there is increased expression of IL-10 which is proved by clearly increased spontaneous production of IL-10 by AD monocytes in vitro.[41,42] This IL 10 has suppressive effect on Th1 cell proliferation and function. In vitro studies also indicate that monocytes might cause the decreased IFN-γ production by T cells from patients with AD.[43] In 1990, Reinhold et al.[44] demonstrated reduced interferon gamma (IFN-γ) production by peripheral blood mononuclear cells of patients with AD. Subsequent studies showed increased interleukin (IL)-4 production by atopic T cells in vitro.[45,46]

Dendritic Cells

Langerhans cells (LCs) have a possible pathogenic role in AD. Studies show that increased numbers of these cells are seen in chronic AD lesions.[47] Bruynzeel–Koomen et al.[48] later demonstrated that more of these cells carried cytophilic IgE antibodies. Those observations led to the demonstration of FcεRII (CD23) expression and to the demonstration of FcεRI high-affinity IgE receptors on LCs and monocytes from patients with AD.[49] The lesional LCs are hyperstimulatory for autologous T cells[50] and that aeroallergen-specific IgE can increase the antigen-presenting function of LCs in patients with AD.[51] Hence, it is clear that IgE might contribute to the abnormal cellular, immune and eczematous responses seen in AD.

EOSINOPHILS

That AD patients have increased circulating eosinophils is well known;[52] but intact eosinophils are sparse in AD lesional tissue. Hence, the exact role of eosinophils in the pathogenesis of AD was not clear for a long time. Despite a paucity of intact infiltrating eosinophils, eosinophil granule proteins are prominently deposited in lesions of AD though there are not many infiltrating eosinophils seen and eosinophil granule proteins are also elevated in the peripheral blood of patients with AD. Based on these findings various studies have reported relationships between eosinophils and AD disease activity, summarized in part in a review.[53] These studies showed that blood eosinophil counts roughly correlated with disease severity, although many patients with severe disease showed normal peripheral blood eosinophil counts. This has been explained by the observation that the patients with normal eosinophil counts were mainly those with AD alone while those with increased peripheral blood eosinophils have severe AD and concomitant respiratory allergies.[54] The altered expression of TH2 cytokines, that is, increased IL-4, IL-5, and IL-13 and decreased IFN-γ expression, observed in patients with AD is the result of increased IgE and eosinophilia.

ROLE OF INFECTIOUS AGENTS AND SUPERANTIGENS IN AD

Infectious agents play a major role in exacerbation of existing AD. AD can be exacerbated by fungal, bacterial and viral skin infections (including herpes simplex, vaccinia, warts, molluscum contagiosum and papillomavirus) apart from food and inhalant allergens. On the other hand, superficial fungal infections, such as tinea caused by *Trichophyton rubrum*,[55] appear to occur more frequently in atopic individuals. Recurrence of dermatophyte infections has also been documented to coincide with flaring of AD. *Malassezia furfur* is a lipophilic yeast commonly present in the seborrheic areas of the skin, and IgE antibodies against *M. furfur* are commonly found in patients with AD, most frequently in those with head and neck dermatitis.[56] The reduction in severity of AD after treatment with antifungal agents indicates the potential importance of *M. furfur* and dermatophyte infections in AD. The potential importance of *M. furfur* and other dermatophyte infections is supported by the reduction in severity of AD after treatment with antifungal agents, such as ketoconazole, in patients with these infections. *Staphylococcus aureus* which is found in only 5% of normal subjects is found in more than 90% of AD skin lesions,[57] and thus many studies have examined the contribution of *S. aureus* colonization and infection to the severity of AD. The density of *S. aureus* on inflamed AD lesions without clinical superinfection can reach up to 10^7 colony-forming units per square centimeter.[58] One method by which *S. aureus* exacerbates or maintains skin inflammation in AD is by secreting a group of toxins known to act as superantigens (enterotoxins A and B, and toxic shock syndrome toxin-1). They stimulate marked activation of T cells and macrophages.[59-61] Most patients with AD have specific IgE antibodies directed against the staphylococcal toxins found on their skin. There is a correlation between the severity of AD and the presence of level of IgE antisuperantigens.[60-61] Superantigens secreted by *S. aureus* have also been shown to induce corticosteroid resistance suggesting that several mechanisms exist by which superantigens could aggravate the severity of AD. In AD, staphylococcal superantigens secreted at the skin surface could penetrate inflamed skin and stimulate epidermal macrophages or Langerhans cells to produce IL-1, TNF, and IL-12. Local production of IL-1 and TNF induces the expression of E-selectin on vascular endothelium, allowing an initial influx of CLA+ memory/effector cells. Local secretion of IL-12 could increase CLA expression on those T cells activated by allergen or superantigen, and thereby increase the efficiency of T-cell recirculation to the skin. IL-12 secreted by toxin-stimulated Langerhans cells (which migrate to skin-associated lymph nodes and serve as antigen-presenting cells) could up-regulate the expression of CLA and influence the functional profile of virgin T cells activated by the toxins, thereby creating additional skin-homing memory-effector T cells.

BARRIER DYSFUNCTION IN ATOPIC DERMATITIS

The stratum corneum constitutes the main barrier for the diffusion of substances through the skin. It consists of corneocytes and intercellular lipids, especially ceramides, sterols, and free fatty acids. Traditionally, the structure of the stratum corneum is linked to a brick wall in which flattened keratinocytes in the corneal layer form the bricks, and lipid lamellae composed of ceramides, cholesterol, and free fatty acids constitute the mortar. The plasma membrane of keratinocytes is replaced by an insoluble protein structure known as the cornified protein envelope, which serves as a scaffold for lipid attachment. The mostly proteinaceous cornified envelope is made up of filaggrin, loricrin, trichohyalin, involucrin, small proline-rich proteins, hornerin, and keratin intermediate filaments, which are crosslinked by transglutaminases. Attached to the outer surface of this cornified envelope is a lipid layer referred to as the corneocyte lipid envelope. Ceramides constitute more than 50% of this intercellular lipid layer. For synthesis of ceramides, precursors sphingomyelin and glucosylceramide contained in lammelar granules are released into the intercellular space and get converted to ceramide. Ceramides are involved in the water-holding properties and thus majorly contribute to the stratum corneum barrier function. There is an impaired barrier function of the stratum corneum in patients with AD. This is due to the dry skin, increased transepidermal water loss and reduction in ceramides in the epidermis, especially ceramide-1. The reduction in ceramide is due to multiple factors as follows:

- There is an abnormal expression of sphingomyelin deacylase, which hydrolyzes sphingomyelin to yield sphingo-phosphorylcholine rather than ceramide.[62-64] This leads to a deleterious effects on the function of the stratum corneum[65]
- The bacterial skin flora obtained from both lesional and nonlesional skin of patients with AD secrete ceramidase which metabolizes ceramide to sphingosine and fatty acids and further adding to the deficiency of ceramide in the stratum corneum).[66]

"Outside-Inside-Outside" Hypothesis (Fig. 2.1)

Whether the defect in cutaneous permeability barrier is a consequence of inflammation[67] or the xerosis and/or permeability barrier abnormality could drive disease activity in AD and other inflammatory dermatoses constitutes the "outside-inside" hypothesis.[68] It is explained in the figure given below. In the ' outside - inside - outside ' model of AD proposed by Elias in 2008, cytokines released as a consequence of barrier damage by environmental agents further injure the barrier creating a self - perpetuating cycle of skin barrier damage and inflammation.[69]

Three proposed sites for therapeutic intervention in AD. At least 3 pathogenic mechanisms contribute to the pathogenesis of AD and therapies are accordingly aimed at them.[70]

As per one theory, barrier dysfunction could be driving disease activity because it fluctuates in relation to disease activity. The underlying SC lipid abnormality in AD is neither addressed properly nor corrected by moisturizers and water in oil emollients. Moreover, improperly formulated moisturizers and emollients can aggravate permeability barrier abnormalities and therefore instead of helping, they could both sustain preexisting disease and exacerbate previously quiescent dermatoses. Ideally as per studies, topical mixtures of the 3 key SC lipids comprise ceramide, cholesterol and free fatty acids, should be applied in optimized proportions (i.e. a 3:1:1 molar ratio) to accelerate barrier repair after a variety of external, acute, or sustained perturbations of the skin barrier.[71-73] Prevention strategies in AD using allergen avoidance have not been consistently effective due to its impracticality. According to a recent study, correcting skin barrier defects from birth may prevent AD onset or moderate disease

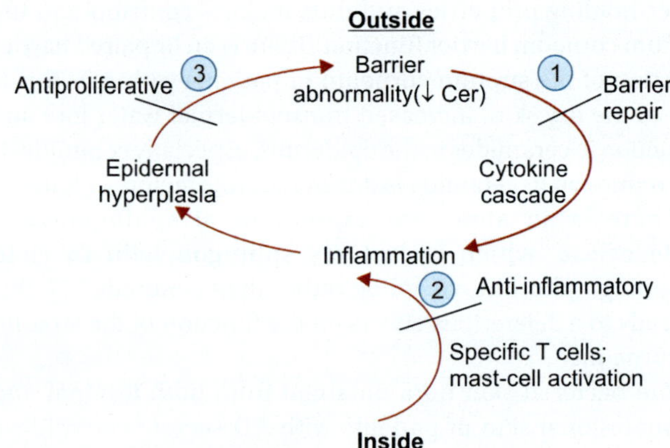

Fig. 2.1 Hypothesis for atopic dermatitis

severity. Skin barrier repair from birth thus represents a novel and feasible approach to AD prevention.[74]

Role of Tight Junctions in AD

Stratum corneum is the most important structure responsible for the barrier to water loss from the skin. However, studies indicate tight junctions, which occur in the stratum granulosum, also play a role. These tight junctions act like gates regulating entry and exit of water and other solutes through the epidermis. Compromise of this paracellular pathway due to defect in tight junction proteins (namely claudin) also contributes to barrier dysfunction in AD.

ROLE OF SWEAT AND ITS ANTIGENS IN ITCH OF AD

Sweating is a known trigger factor for the itch in AD. It has been suggested that blockage of sweat ducts and its release into the dermis triggers the itch in AD. The sweat of patients with AD has also been shown to contain specific IgE antibodies to inhalant allergens and may play a role in antigen capture. Biofilms of *Staphylococcus epidermidis* in cultures from patients with flexural eczema (similar process accounts for the itch in miliaria). Extracellular polysaccharide substance released from this organism contributes to the itch in AD especially in flexures wherein a milaria-like subclinical pathology may occur.

ROLE OF HISTAMINE AND NEUROPEPTIDES IN AD

Since antihistamines (H1 and H2 blockers) do not relieve pruritus in AD, histamine is not an important mediator for the itch of AD. A third histamine receptor (H3) and a fourth histamine receptor (H4) expressed on numerous immune and inflammatory cells may also be responsible for this itch. There is evidence that there may be alteration of peripheral nerve endings in AD. Higher nerve fiber density in lichenified lesions than in uninvolved skin may be the result of repeated scratching causing mechanical damage to free nerve endings. There appears to be a complex interaction of peripheral nerves, neurotrophic factors, lymphocytes, mast cells, eosinophils, and dendritic cells in areas of AD. Nerve growth factors are consequently seen to be higher in lesional skin of AD patients. Brain-derived neurotrophic factor (BDNF), a growth factor originally identified in the nervous system, is also now known to produced by circulating eosinophils. Levels of BDNF are significantly correlated with disease activity and nocturnal scratching in children with AD.

CONCLUSION

Susceptibility to AD largely depends on genetics. But there is a complex interaction between environmental factors and susceptibility genes resulting in clinical expression of the disorder. Recent increase in prevalence of AD suggests the importance of environmental factors. These environmental immunologic "triggers" differ among individuals and include various foods, airborne allergens, irritants and contactants, hormones, stress, climate, and microorganisms. Multiple triggers can be generally identified in one individual and this profile of triggers may undergo a change with time. AD is most commonly associated with IgE-related mechanisms, and the vast majority of patients with AD exhibit hyperproduction of IgE. Although AD has been characterized as a TH2-type disorder within the TH1/TH2 paradigm, research has revealed that a biphasic response model may account more accurately for the underlying immunologic mechanisms; patients initially exhibit TH2-like immune responses early in the acute stage and switch to a more TH1-like profile as chronic lesions emerge.

REFERENCES

1. Palmer LJ, Burton PR, Faux JA, James AL, Musk AW, Cookson WO. Independent inheritance of serum immunoglobulin E concentrations and airway responsiveness. Am J Respir Crit Care Med. 2000;161:1836-43.
2. Larsen FS, Holm NV, Henningsen K. Atopic dermatitis. A genetic-epidemiologic study in a population-based twin sample. J Am Acad Dermatol. 1986;15:487-94.
3. Schultz LF. Atopic dermatitis: a genetic epidemiologic study in a population-based twin sample. J Am Acad Dermatol. 1993;28:719-23.
4. Bohme M, Wickman M, Lennart NS, Svartengren M, Wahgren C. Family history and risk of atopic dermatitis in children up to 4 years. Clin Exp Allergy. 2003;33:1226-31.
5. Kaufman HS, Frick OL. The development of allergy in infants of allergic parents: A prospective study concerning the role of heredity. Ann Allergy. 1976;37:410-5.
6. Davis SD, Schaller J, Wedgwood RJ. Job's syndrome: recurrent, cold staphylococcal abscesses. Lancet 1966;1:1013-5.
7. Borges WG, Hertsley T, Carey JC, Petrak BA, Hill HR. The face of Job. J Pediatr. 1998;133:303-5.
8. Judge MR, Morgan G, Harper JI. A clinical and immunological study of Netherton's syndrome. Br J Dermatol. 1994;131:615-21.
9. Cookson WO, Ubhi B, Lawrence R, et al. Genetic linkage of childhood atopic dermatitis to psoriasis susceptibility loci. Nat Genet. 2001;27:372-3.

10. Bradley M, Soderhall C, Luthman H, et al. Susceptibility loci for atopic dermatitis on chromosomes 3, 13, 15, 17 and 18 in a Swedish population. Hum Mol Genet. 2002;11:1539-48.

11. Lee YA, Wahn U, Kehrt R, et al. A major susceptibility locus for atopic dermatitis maps to chromosome 3q21. Nat Genet, 2000; 26:470-3.

12. Haagerup A, Bjerke T, Schiotz PO, et al. Atopic dermatitis—a total genome-scan for susceptibility genes. Acta Derm Venereol. 2004;84:346-52.

13. Mischke D, Korge BP, Marenholz I, Volz A, Ziegler A. Genes encoding structural proteins of epidermal cornification and S100 calcium-binding proteins form a gene complex ("epidermal differentiation complex") on human chromosome 1q21. J Invest Dermatol. 1996;106(5):989-92.

14. Palmer CN, Irvine AD, Terron-Kwiatkowski A, et al. Common loss-of-function variants of the epidermal barrier protein filaggrin are a major predisposing factor for atopic dermatitis. Nat Genet. 2006;38:441-6.

15. Stemmler S, Parwez Q, Petrasch-Parwez E, et al. Two common loss-of-function mutations within the filaggrin gene predispose for early onset of atopic dermatitis. J Invest Dermatol. 2007;127:722-4.

16. Barker JN, Palmer CN, Zhao Y, et al. Null mutations in the filaggrin gene (FLG) determine major susceptibility to early-onset atopic dermatitis that persists into adulthood. J Invest Dermatol. 2007;127:564-7.

17. Candi E, Schmidt R, Melino G. The cornified envelope: A model of cell death in the skin. Nat Rev Mol Cell Biol. 2005;6(4):328-40.

18. Deichmann KA, Heinzmann A, Forster J, et al. Linkage and allelic association of atopy and markers fl anking the IL4-receptor gene. Clin Exp Allergy. 1998;28:151-5.

19. Hershey GK, Friedrich MF, Esswein LA, et al. The association of atopy with a gain-of-function mutation in the alpha subunit of the interleukin-4 receptor. N Engl J Med. 1997;337:1720-5.

20. Kruse S, Japha T, Tedner M, et al. The polymorphisms S503P and Q576R in the interleukin-4 receptor alpha gene are associated with atopy and influence the signal transduction. Immunology. 1999;96:365-71.

21. Sandford AJ, Shirakawa T, Moffatt MF, et al. Localisation of atopy and beta subunit of high-affinity IgE receptor (Fc epsilon RI) on chromosome 11q. Lancet 1993;341:332-4.

22. Nickel RG, Casolaro V, Wahn U, et al. Atopic dermatitis is associated with a functional mutation in the promoter of the C-C chemokine RANTES. J Immunol. 2000;164:1612-6.

23. Walley AJ, Chavanas S, Moffatt MF, et al. Gene polymorphism in Netherton and common atopic disease. Nat Genet. 2001;29:175-8.

24. Kato A, Fukai K, Oiso N, et al. Association of SPINK5 gene polymorphisms with atopic dermatitis in the Japanese population. Br J Dermatol. 2003;148:665-9.
25. Nishio Y, Noguchi E, Shibasaki M, et al. Association between polymorphisms in the SPINK5 gene and atopic dermatitis in the Japanese. Genes Immun. 2003;4:515-7.
26. Dold S, Wjst M, von Mutius E, et al. Genetic risk for asthma, allergic rhinitis, and atopic dermatitis. Arch Dis Child. 1992;67:1018-22.
27. Ruiz RG, Kemeny DM, Price JF. Higher risk of infantile atopic dermatitis from maternal atopy than from paternal atopy. Clin Exp Allergy. 1992;22:762-6.
28. Strachan DP. Hay fever, hygiene, and household size. BMJ. 1989;299:1259-60.
29. Matricardi PM, Rosmini F, Riondino S, et al. Exposure to foodborne and orofecal microbes versus airborne viruses in relation to atopy and allergic asthma: epi-demiological study. BMJ. 2000;320:412-7.
30. Thepen T, Langeveld-Wildschut G, Bihari IC, Van Wichen DF, Van Reijsen FC, Mudde GC. Biphasic response against aeroallergen in atopic dermatitis showing a switch from an initial TH2 response to a TH1response in situ: an immunocytochemical study. J Allergy Clin Immunol. 1996;97:828-37.
31. Hanifin JM, Chan SC. Monocyte phosphodiesterase abnormalities and dysregulation of lymphocyte function in atopic dermatitis. J Invest Dermatol. 1995;105(suppl):84S-88S.
32. Hamid Q, Boguniewicz M, Leung DYM. Differential in situ cytokine gene expression in acute vs. chronic atopic dermatitis. J Clin Invest. 1994;94:870-6.
33. Hamid Q, Naseer T, Minshall EM, Song YL, Boguniewicz M, Leung DYM. In vivo expression of IL-12 and IL-13 in atopic dermatitis. J Allergy Clin Immunol. 1996;98:225-31.
34. Picker LJ, Martin RJ, Trumble A, Newman LS, Collins PA, Bergstresser PR, et al. Differential expression of lymphocyte homing receptors by human memory/effector T cells in pulmonary versus cutaneous immune effector sites. Eur J Immunol. 1994;24:1269-77.
35. Ohman S, Johansson SG. Immunoglobulins in atopic dermatitis. Acta Derm Venereol (Stockh). 1974;54:193.
36. Jones HE, Inouye JC, McGerity JL, Lewis CW. Atopic disease and serum immunoglobulin-E. Br J Dermatol. 1975;92:17-25.
37. Peterson RD, Page AR, Good RA. Wheal and erythema allergy in patients with agammaglobulinemia. J Allergy. 1966;33:406-11.
38. Hanifin JM, Lobitz WC. Newer concepts of atopic dermatitis. Arch Dermatol. 1977;113:663-7.
39. Elliott ST, Hanifin JM. Delayed cutaneous hypersensitivity and lymphocyte transformation: dissociation in atopic dermatitis. Arch Dermatol. 1979;115:36-9.

40. Zachary CB, Allen MH, MacDonald DM. In situ quantification of T-lymphocyte subsets and Langerhans cells in the inflammatory infiltrate of atopic eczema. Br J Dermatol. 1985;112:149-56.
41. Ohmen JD, Hanifin JM, Nickoloff BJ, Rea TH, Wyzykowski R, Kim J. Overexpression of IL-10 in atopic dermatitis: contrasting cytokine patterns with delayed-type hypersensitivity reactions. J Immunol. 1995;154:1956-63.
42. Asadullah K, Sterry W, Stephanek K, Jasulaitis D, Leupold M, Audring H. IL-10 is a key cytokine in psoriasis: proof of principle by IL-10 therapy: a new therapeutic approach. J Clin Invest. 1998;101:783-94.
43. Chan SC, Kim J-W, Henderson WR Jr, Hanifin JM. Altered prostaglandin E2 regulation of cytokine production in atopic dermatitis. J Immunol. 1993;151:3345-52.
44. Reinhold U, Wehrmann W, Kukel S, Kreysel HW. Recombinant interferon-γ in severe atopic dermatitis. Lancet. 1990;1:1282.
45. Jujo KH, Renz J, Abe EW, Leung DY. Decreased interferon-gamma and increased interleukin 4 production in atopic dermatitis promotes IgE synthesis. J Allergy Clin Immunol. 1992;90:323-31.
46. Chan SC, Li S-H, Hanifin JM. Increased interleukin 4 production by atopic mononuclear leukocytes correlates with increased cyclic AMP-PDE activity and is reversible by PDE inhibition. J Invest Dermatol. 1993;100:681-4.
47. Uno H, Hanifin JM. Langerhans cells in acute and chronic epidermal lesions of atopic dermatitis, observed by L-Dopa histofluorescence, glycol methacrylate thin section, and electron microscopy. J Invest Dermatol. 1980;75:52-60.
48. Bruynzeel-Koomen CA, van Wichen DF, Toonstra J, Berrens L, Bruynzeel PL. The presence of IgE molecules on epidermal Langerhans cells in patients with atopic dermatitis. Arch Dermatol Res. 1986;278:199-205.
49. Bieber T, de la Salle C, Wollenberg A, Chizzonite R, Hakimi J, et al. Human Langerhans cells express the high-affinity receptor for immunoglobulin E. J Exp Med. 1992;175:1285-90.
50. Taylor RS, Baadsgaard O, Hammerberg C, Cooper KD. Hyperstimulatory CD1a+CD1b+CD36+ Langerhans cells are responsible for increased autologous T lymphocyte reactivity to lesional epidermal cells of patients with atopic dermatitis. J-Immunol. 1991;147:3794-802.
51. Mudde GC, Van Reijsen FC, Boland GJ, De Gast GC, Bruijnkeel PL, Bruijnkeel-Koomen CA. Allergen presentation by epidermal Langerhans cells from patients with atopic dermatitis is mediated by IgE. Immunology. 1990;69:335-41.
52. Rajka G. Atopic dermatitis. Major Probl Dermatol. 1975;3:42.
53. Kapp A. The role of eosinophils in the pathogenesis of atopic dermatitis: eosinophil granule proteins as markers of disease activity. Allergy. 1993;48:1-5.

54. Uehara M, Izukura R, Sawai T. Blood eosinophilia in atopic dermatitis. Clin Exp Dermatol. 1990;15:264-6.
55. Jones HE, Reinhardt JH, Rinaldi MG. A clinical, mycological and immunological survey for dermatophytosis. Arch Dermatol. 1973;107:217-22.
56. Kieffer M, Bergbrant I-M, Faergemann J, Jemec GB, Ottevanger V, Stahl Skov P, et al. Immune reactions to Pityrosporum ovalein adult patients with atopic and seborrheic dermatitis. J Am Acad Dermatol. 1990;22:739-42.
57. Leyden JE, Marples RR, Kligman AM. *Staphylococcus aureus* in the lesions of atopic dermatitis. Br J Dermatol. 1974;90:525-30.
58. Hauser C, Wuethrich B, Matter L, Wilhelm J, Sonnabend W, Schopfer K. *Staphylococcus aureus* skin colonization in atopic dermatitis patients. Dermatologica. 1985;170:35-9.
59. Bunikowski R, Mielke MEA, Skarabis H, Worm M, Anagnostopoulos I, Kolde G, et al. Evidence for a disease-promoting effect of *Staphylococcus aureus*-derived exotoxins in atopic dermatitis. J Allergy Clin Immunol. 2000;105:814-9.
60. Nomura I, Tanaka K, Tomita H, Katsunuma T, Ohya Y, Ikeda N, et al. Evaluation of the staphylococcal exotoxins and their specific IgE in childhood atopic dermatitis. J Allergy Clin Immunol. 1999;104:441-6.
61. Bunikowski R, Mielke M, Skarabis H, Herz U, Bergmann RL, Wahn U, et al. Prevalence and role of serum IgE antibodies to the *Staphylococcus aureus*-derived superantigens SEA and SEB in children with atopic dermatitis. J Allergy Clin Immunol. 1999;103:119-24.
62. Imokawa G, Abe A, Jin K, Migaki Y, Kawashima M, Hidano A. Decreased levels of ceramides in stratum corneum of atopic dermatitis: An etiologic factor in atopic dry skin? J Invest Dermatol. 1991;96:523-6.
63. Dinardo A, Wertz P, Giannetti A, Seidenari S. Ceramide and cholesterol composition of the skin of patients with atopic dermatitis. Acta Derm Venereol (Stockh). 1998;78:27-30.
64. Breck O, Abrek D, Ring J, Hoppe U, Vietzke J-P, Wolber R, et al. Two ceramide subfractions detectable in CER (AS) position by HPTLC in skin surface lipids of nonlesional skin of atopic eczema. J Invest Dermatol. 1999;113:894-900.
65. Murata Y, Ogata J, Higaki Y, Kawashima M, Yada Y, Higuchi K, et al. Abnormal expression sphingomyelin acylase in atopic dermatitis: an etiologic factor for ceramide deficiency? J Invest Dermatol. 1996;106:1242-9.
66. Ohnishi Y, Okino N, Ito M, Irryama S. Ceramidase activity in bacterial skin flora as a possible cause of ceramide deficiency in atopic dermatitis. Clin Diagn Lab Immunol. 1999;6:101-4.
67. Leung DY. Atopic dermatitis: new insights and opportunities for therapeutic intervention. J Allergy Clin Immunol. 2000;105:860-76.

68. Elias PM, Wood LC, Feingold KR. Epidermal pathogenesis of inflammatory dermatoses. Am J Contact Dermatitis. 1999;10:119-26.
69. Elias PM, Steinhoff M. 'Outside – to – inside ' (and now back to 'outside') pathogenic mechanisms in atopic dermatitis. J Invest Dermatol. 2008;128;(5):1067-70).
70. Chamlin SL, Kao J, Frieden IJ, Sheu MY, et al. Ceramide-dominant barrier repair lipids alleviate childhood atopic dermatitis: Changes in barrier function provide a sensitive indicator of disease activity. J Am Acad Dermatol. 2002;47:198-208.
71. Mao-Qiang M, Brown BE, Wu-Pong S, Feingold KR, Elias PM. Exogenous nonphysiologic vs physiologic lipids. Divergent mechanisms for correction of permeability barrier dysfunction. Arch Dermatol. 1995;131:809-16.
72. Man MM, Feingold KR, Thornfeldt CR, Elias PM. Optimization of physiological lipid mixtures for barrier repair. J Invest Dermatol. 1996;106:1096-101.
73. Yang L, Mao-Qiang M, Taljebini M, Elias PM, Feingold KR. Topical stratum corneum lipids accelerate barrier repair after tape stripping, solvent treatment and some but not all types of detergent treatment. Br J Dermatol. 1995;133:679-85.
74. Simpson EL, Berry TM, Brown PA, Hanifin JN. A pilot study of emollient therapy for the primary prevention of atopic dermatitis. J Am Acad Dermatol. 2010;63:587-93.

Clinical Manifestations of Atopic Dermatitis

Pranjal Ahire, Satish Udare

Atopic Dermatitis (AD) is a chronic, itchy, fluctuating disease, typically begins during infancy with age of onset of 2–6 months in majority of patients, but it may occur at any age. It is one of the most common skin disorders in developed countries, affecting approximately 20% of children and 1–3% of adults.[1]

It is slightly more common in boys than girls.[2] It presents with range of common clinical features enlisted in Table 3.1.

The diagnosis of AD based on constellation of signs and symptoms.

There is no laboratory "gold standard" for the diagnosis of AD.

Hanifin and Rajka for the first time proposed a systematic approach towards the standardization of the diagnosis of AD by incorporating three major/basic and 23 minor features. They suggested that a diagnosis of AD can be established if three of the major and three of the minor criteria are present.[3]

MAJOR/BASIC FEATURES

- Pruritus
- *Typical morphology and distribution:* Flexural lichenification or linearity in adults, facial and extensor involvement in infants and children
- Chronic or chronically-relapsing dermatitis
- Personal or family history of atopy (asthma, AR, AD).

Pruritus in AD is main cardinal symptom, and is essential for diagnosis. and the disease was described as 'itch that rashes' it is severe, episodic, mainly in night and disturbs patient and surrounding people, caretakers and results in poor QOL.

Table 3.1: Clinical features of atopic dermatitis

- Pruritus
- Macular erythema/papules/papulovesicles on face and extensors in infants and young children Fig 3.1
- Eczematous lesions with crusting Fig 3.2
- Lichenification in flexural areas in older children (Figs 3.3 to 3.5)
- Excoriations Fig 3.6
- Secondary infections Fig 3.7
- Dryness of skin Fig 3.8
- Chronic or chronically-relapsing dermatitis. (Fig 3.9)

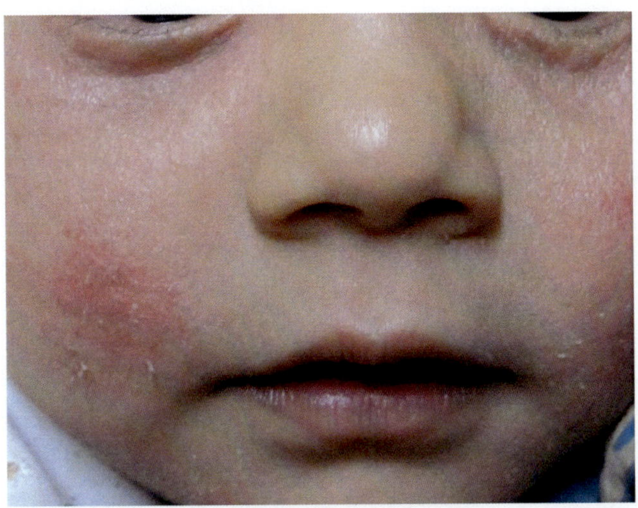

Fig. 3.1: Facial lesions in infant

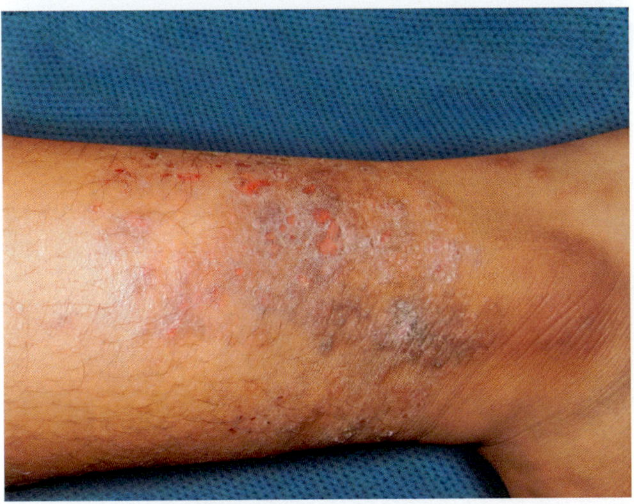

Fig. 3.2: Eczematous lesions with crusting on legs

The itch leads to more inflammation, more scratching, more thickening and lichenification and continues the cycle—the so called 'itch scratch cycle'. Most patients are compulsively scratching without their knowledge and exacerbate their disease. The typical morphology consist of acute, subacute or chronic eczematous rash. Acute eczema shows signs of acute inflammation mainly vesiculation, oozing, erythema and crusting which is mainly seen in infantile phase (Fig. 3.1), in subacute stage the vesiculation is less but scaling, crusting and thickening of skin becomes evident. Chronic form mainly seen in childhood and adult phase. The skin shows lichenification with increased skin markings, few scratch marks and crusting.

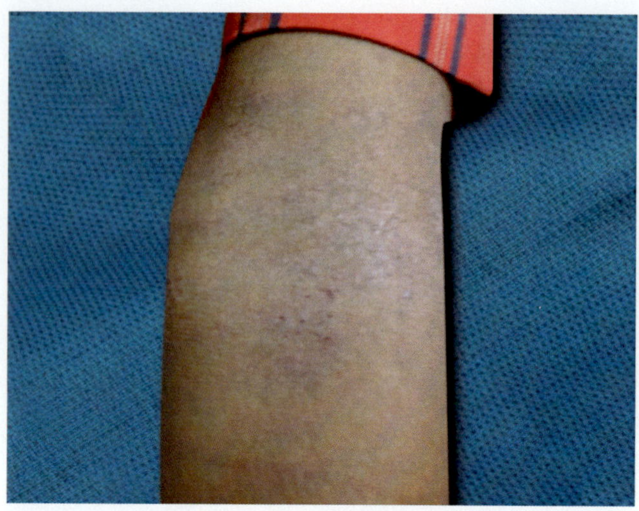

Fig. 3.3: Lichenification in antecubital fossae

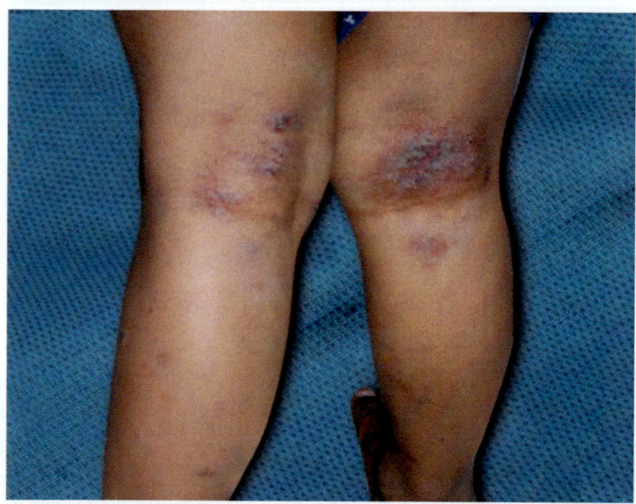

Fig. 3.4: Lichenification in popliteal fossae

The disease has relapsing nature and may present intermittently with acute spread with papulovesicular eruptions all over body but sometimes erupts preferentially only in specific areas.

MINOR OR LESS-CHARACTERISTIC FEATURES

- Xerosis (Fig. 3.8)
- Ichthyosis (Fig. 3.10) palmar hyperlinearity (Fig. 3.11), keratosis pilaris (Fig. 3.12)
- Immediate (type 1) skin test reactivity
- Elevated serum IgE

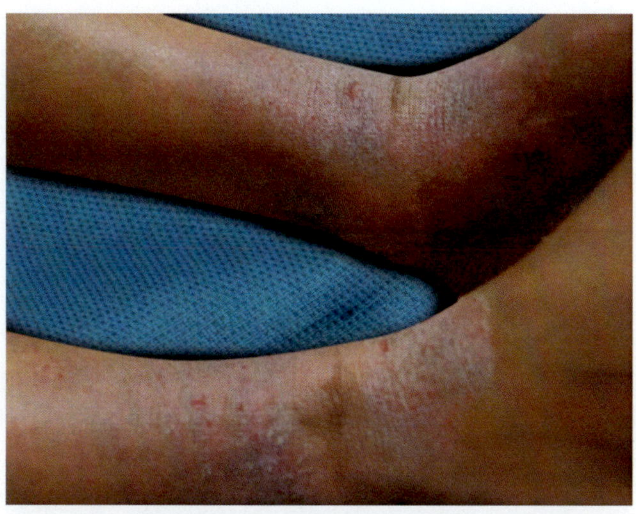

Fig. 3.5: Lichenification on ankle area

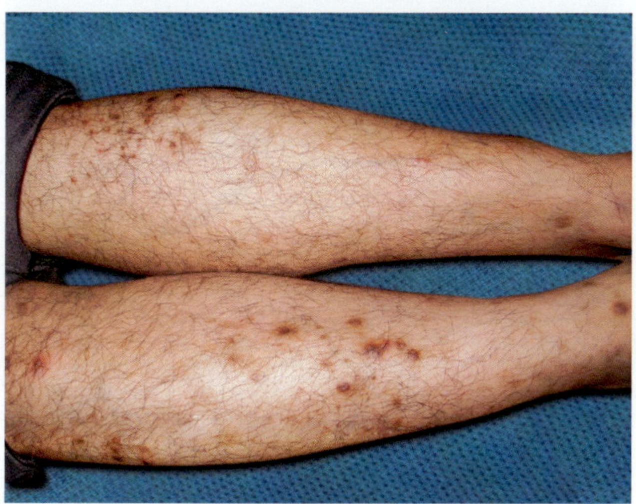

Fig. 3.6: Excoriations

- Early age at onset
- Tendency towards cutaneous infections (especially *S. aureus* and herpes simplex)/impaired cell-mediated immunity (Fig. 3.13)
- Tendency towards nonspecific hand or foot dermatitis (Fig. 3.14)
- Nipple eczema (Fig. 3.15)
- Cheilitis (Fig. 3.16, 3.17)
- Recurrent conjunctivitis
- Dennie–Morgan infraorbital folds (Fig. 3.18)
- Keratoconus

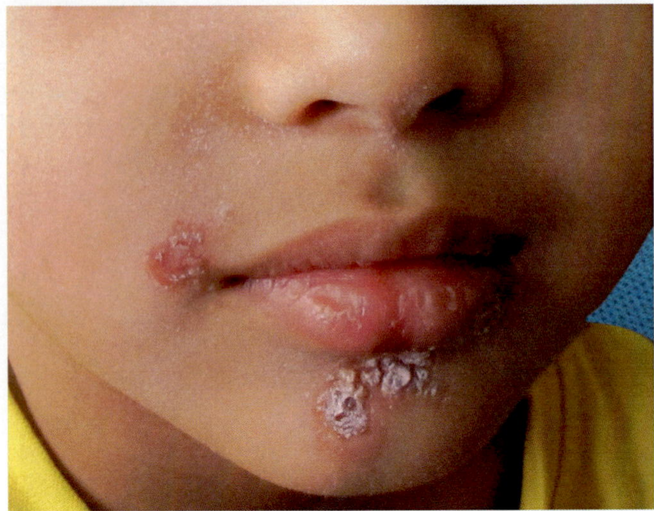

Fig. 3.7: Secondary infections

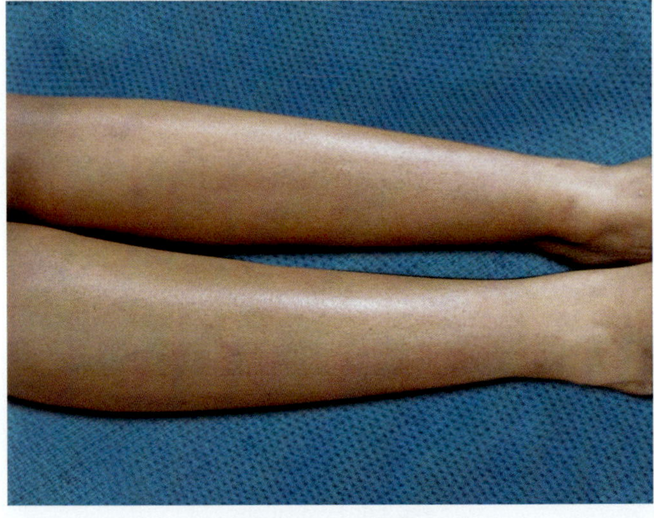

Fig. 3.8: Dry scaly skin of legs

- Anterior subcapsular cataracts
- Orbital darkening
- Facial pallor/facial erythema
- Pityriasis alba (Fig. 3.19)
- Anterior neck folds (Fig. 3.20)
- Itch when sweating
- Intolerance to wool or lipid solvents
- Follicular accentuation and dermatitis (Fig. 3.21, 3.22)
- Food intolerance
- Course influenced by environmental/emotional factors
- White dermographism/delayed blanch.

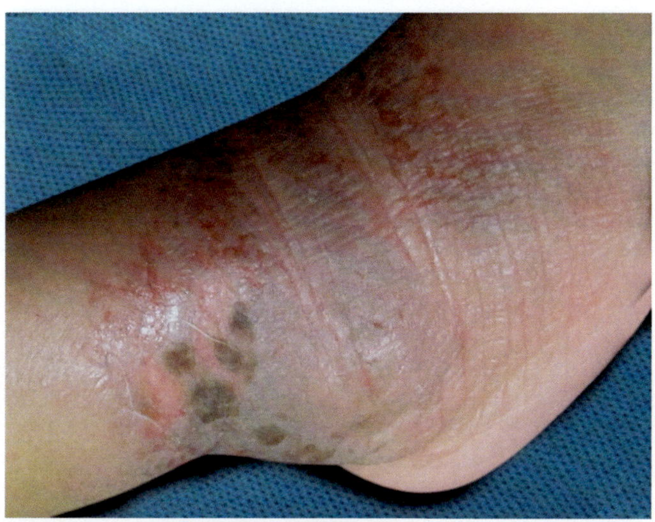

Fig. 3.9: Chronic relapsing lesions on legs

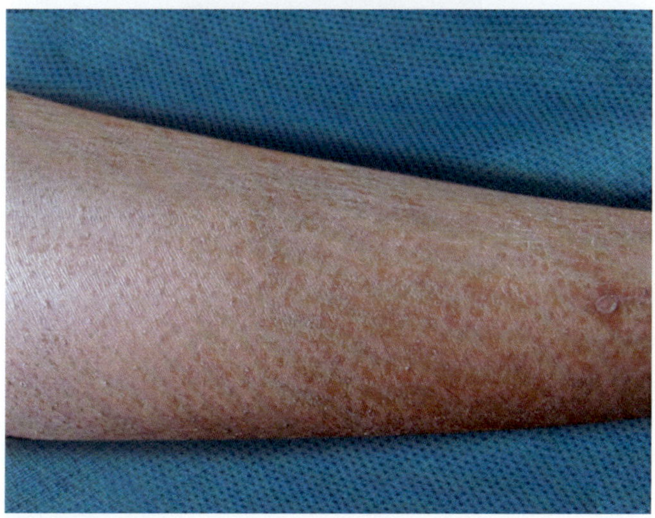

Fig. 3.10: Ichthyosis

Atopic Diathesis consists of presence of AD, allergic rhinitis and asthma.

Atopic march refers to natural history of atopic or allergic manifestations characterized by typical sequence of clinical symptoms and conditions that occur in certain age period and persist over a number of years. Atopic dermatitis affect infants and young children frequently, asthma affects older children and pollen allergy predominantly affects adolescents. This characteristic sequence of events is known as "atopic march". Some of the features become prominent whereas others diminish or disappear over a period of time. Usually symptoms of AD precede allergic rhinitis or asthma.[4]

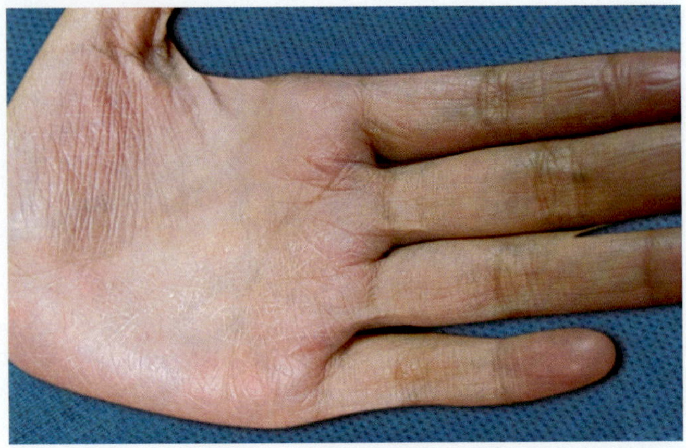

Fig. 3.11: Palmar hyperlinearity

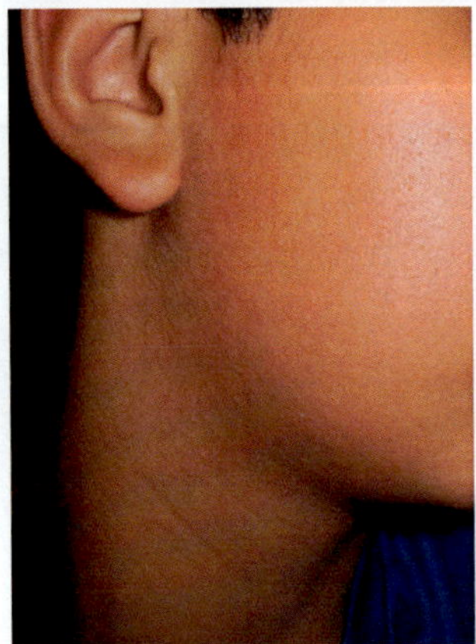

Fig. 3.12: Keratosis pilaris

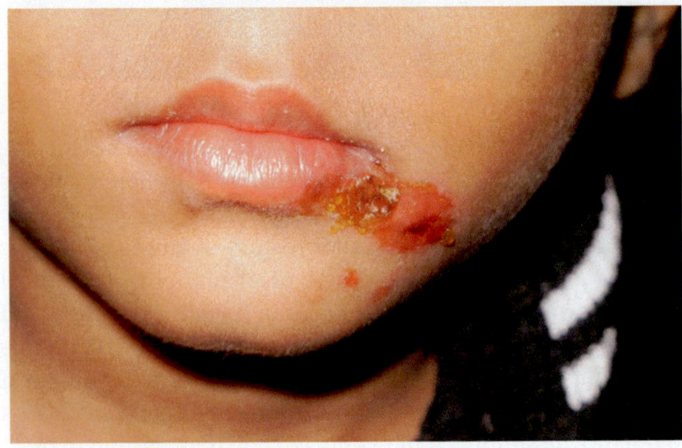

Fig. 3.13: Impetigo in child around mouth

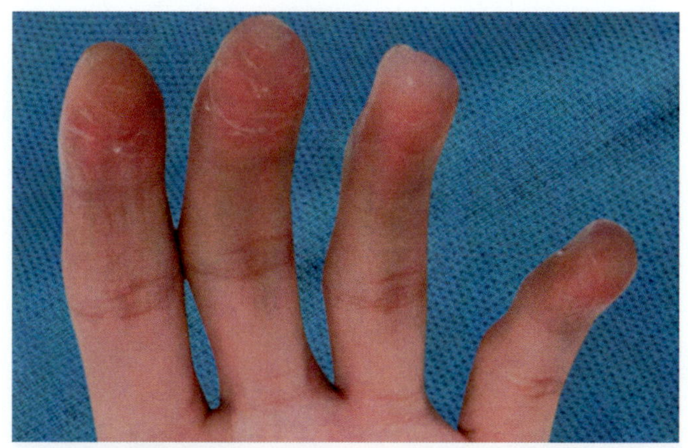

Fig. 3.14: Hand dermatitis at the tip of fingers

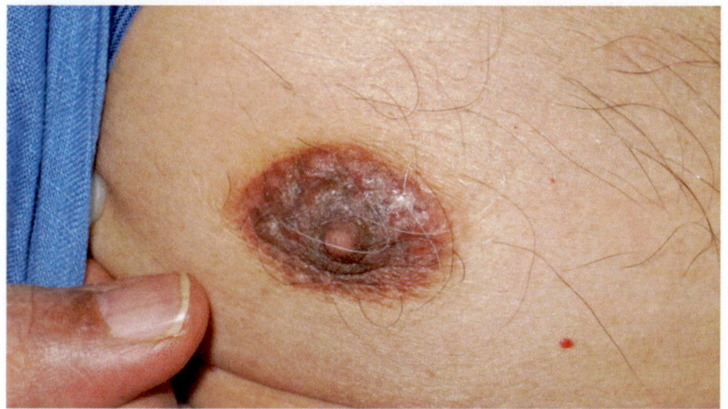

Fig. 3.15: Nipple eczema

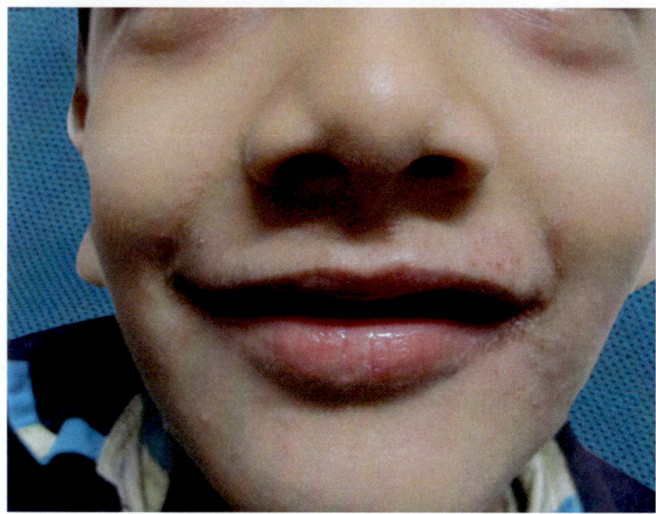

Fig. 3.16: Cheilitis

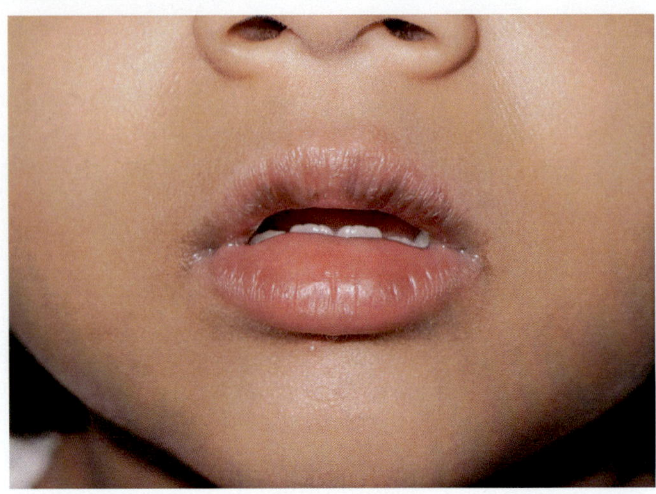

Fig. 3.17: Cheilitis

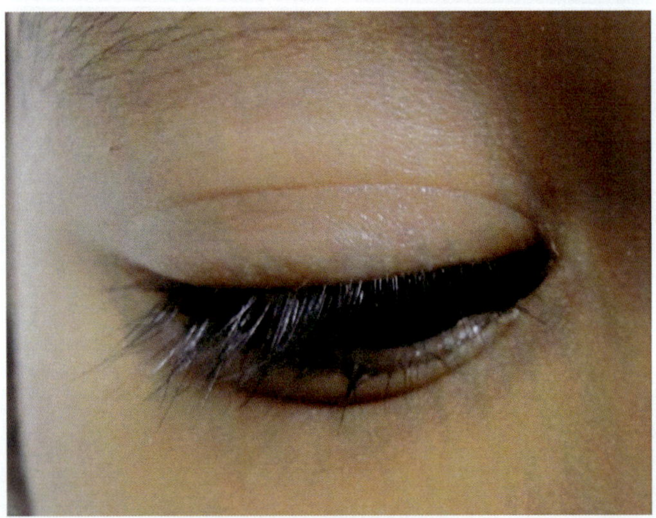

Fig 3.18: Dennie–Morgan fold

Atopic dermatitis is intensely pruritic condition, itching precedes the appearance of lesions hence, it is described as "itch that rashes".

Atopic Dermatitis can be divided into 3 stages: Infantile AD, occurring from 2 months to 2 years of age; childhood AD, from 2 to 10 Years, and adolescent/adult AD.

Pruritus is the major feature in all three stages.

INFANTILE AD

It occurs from 2 months to 2 years of age. Around fifty percent of cases of AD are seen in first year of life. Lesions in infancy

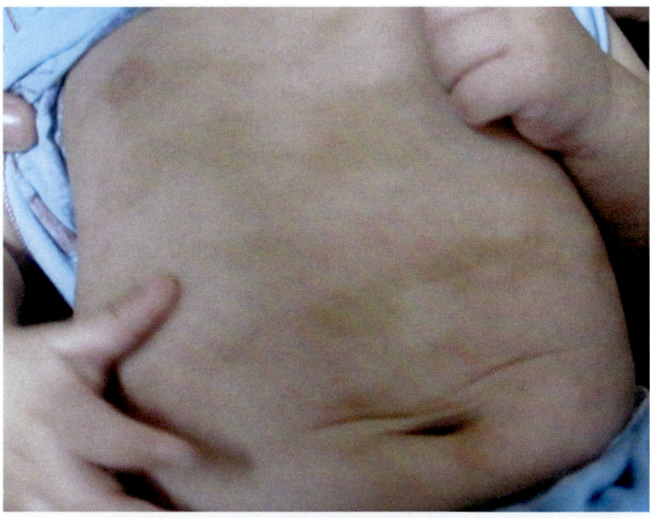

Fig 3.19: Pityriasis alba

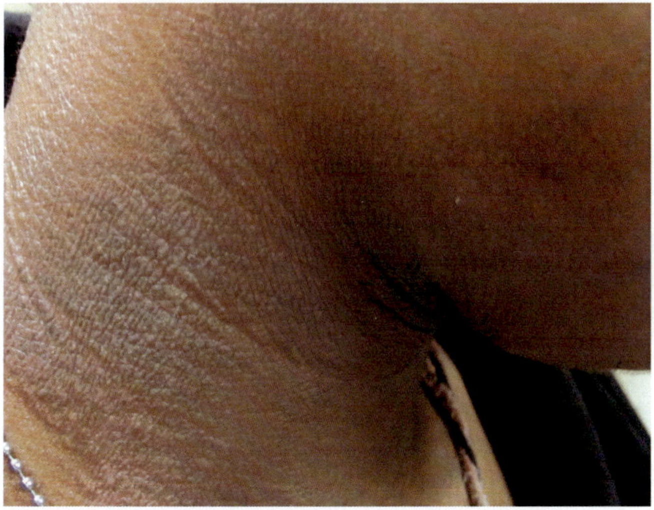

Fig. 3.20: Invovement of anterior neck fold

usually start on face (Fig. 3.23) but they may involve other areas also (Fig. 3.24). Usually infantile AD begins as erythema and scaling of cheeks which later extends to involve scalp, neck, and forehead, wrists[11] and extensor extremities[12] when the child starts crawling. Diaper area is usually spared.[14] Also spared areas are nose and paranasal areas giving the so called "headlight sign". Lesions consist of erythema, papules which are intensely pruritic with exudates, crusting, secondary infection[15] due to chronic rubbing and scratching. Eyelid dermatitis sets in later age which may lead to classic Dennie Morgan fold (Fig. 3.18).[16] The course of disease is chronic and fluctuating, varying with

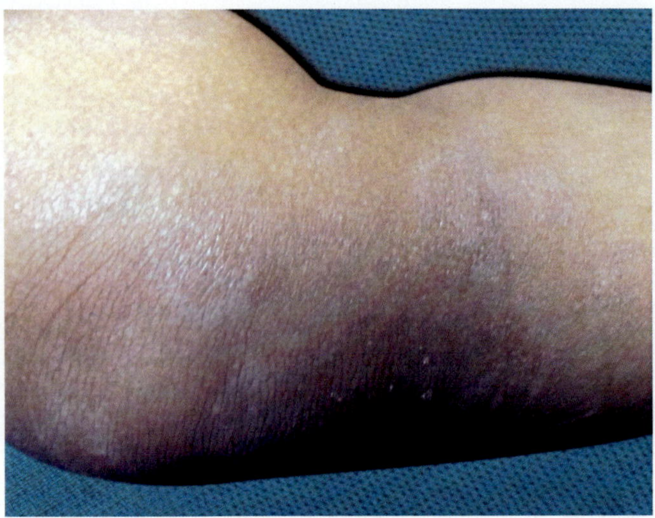

Fig. 3.21: Follicular dermatitis

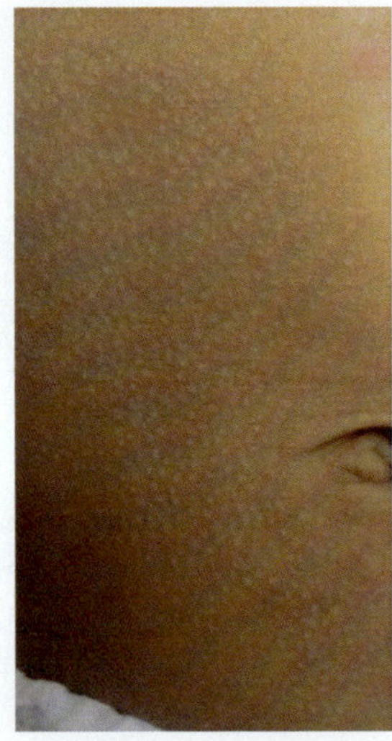

Fig. 3.22: Follicular dermatitis

respiratory infections, immunizations, teething, emotional upsets, climatic changes. Infantile phase persists till the end of second year. Other associated features are mentioned later.

CHILDHOOD AD

In childhood AD lesions tend to be more of lichenified and less exudative. This stage is seen 18–24 months of age till puberty. It involves flexural areas like antecubital fossae, popliteal fossae, flexors of wrists, ankles, sides of neck with characteristic

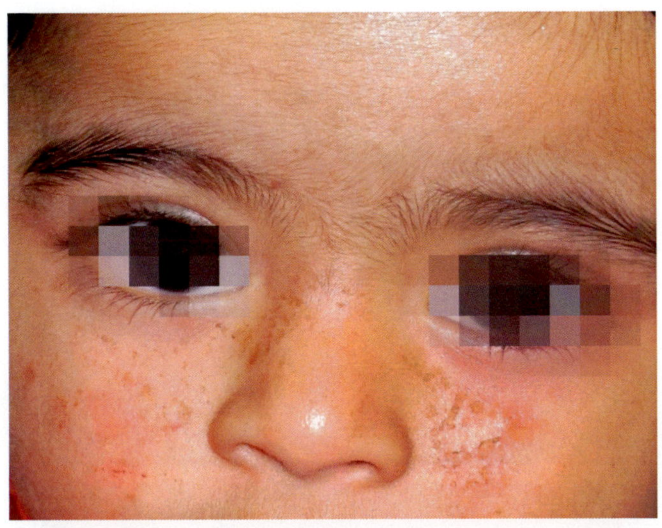

Fig. 3.23: Infantile eczema—lesions on face

reticulate pigmentation of "atopic dirty neck" (Figs 3.25). Axillae are involved infrequently and axillary involvement may be a marker of seborrheic dermatitis. Pruritus is important feature and most clinical features are secondary to chronic rubbing and scratching. There is 'itch-scratch-itch' vicious cycle which leads to lichenification of lesions. Excoriated papules are seen scattered over exposed areas. Pruritus is sometimes severe to disturb sleep of a child leading to poor scholastic performance and psychological disturbances.

Adolescents and adult AD–adult AD begins after puberty and lesions are localized, erythematous, scaly papules, exudative and lichenified (Fig. 3.26). It affects antecubital and popliteal fossae, front and sides of neck, around eyes (Fig. 3.28), forehead and other areas in adolescents (Fig. 3.29). In adults, lesions are localized and may involve hands, nipple and eyelid eczema (Figs 3.18 to 3.25 and 3.27). The hands and fingers are involved frequently with fissures on overlying finger joints, scaling on palms and adjoining fingers (apron sign) (Figs 3.30 to 3.31).[2,6] Sometimes lesions may generalize (Fig. 3.33) with accentuation in flexures. Lesions may be scaly erythematous papules, lichenified or prurigo-like papules (Figs 3.34 and 3.35). Lesions are often excoriated papules, coalesced to form plaques and hyperpigmented in darker skin types (Fig. 3.36). Pruritus often increases in evenings. Flares of AD may be related to acute emotional upsets, stress, anxiety and depression.[5]

Atopic dermatitis in adults improves with age and less common after middle age, but dry skin, exacerbation with specific allergens and environmental condition persists. Photosensitivity (Fig. 3.37), exacerbation (Fig. 3.34) of lesions

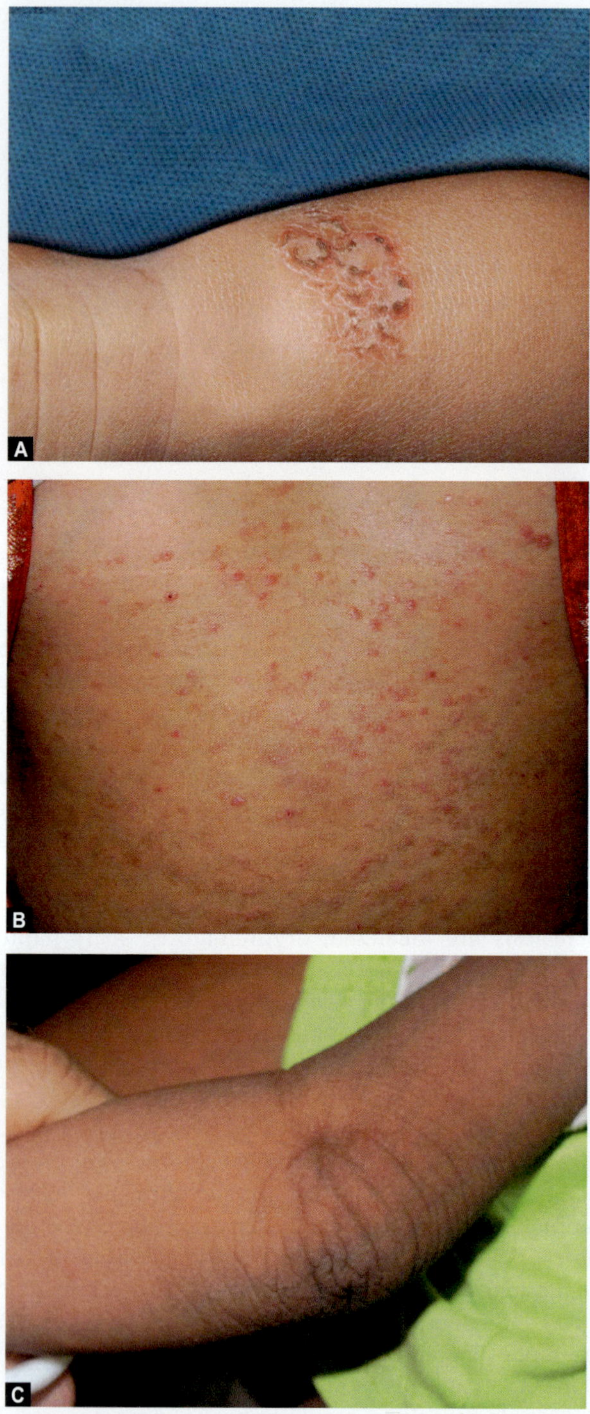

Fig. 3.24A to C: Infantile eczema—lesions on other areas

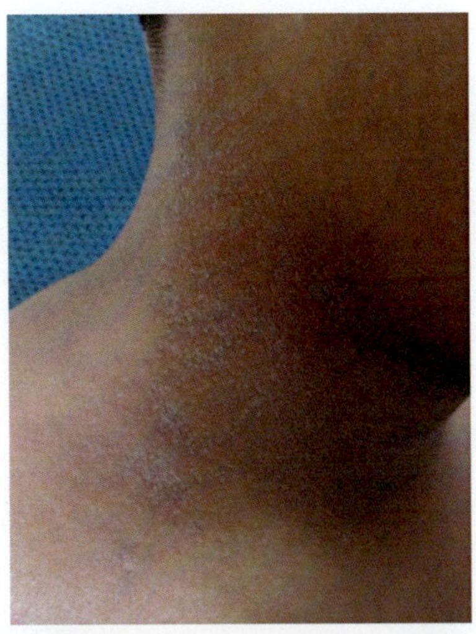

Fig. 3.25: Dirty-neck appearance

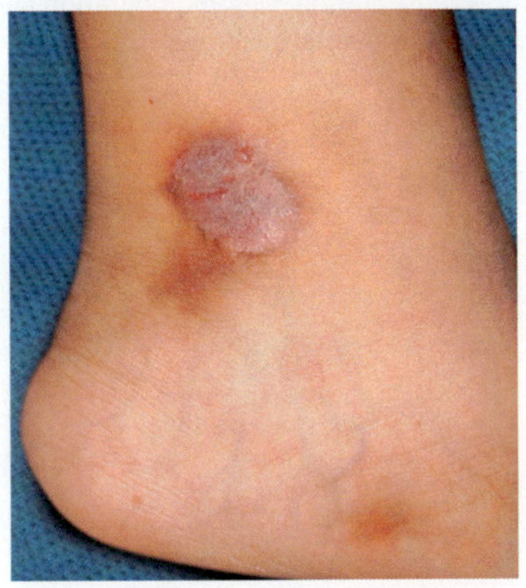

Fig. 3.26: Subacute eczema

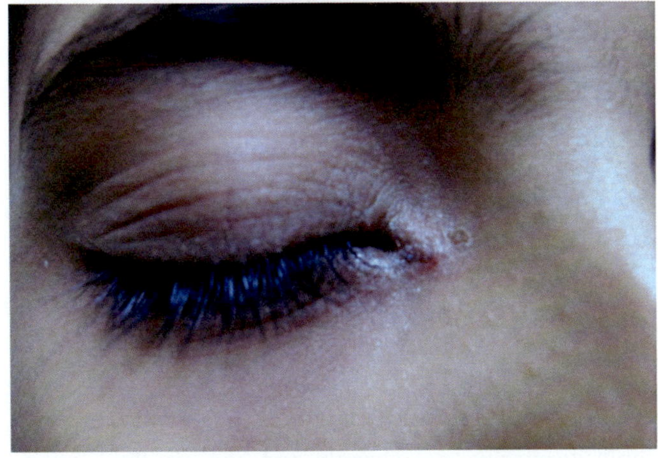

Fig. 3.27: Eyelid eczema

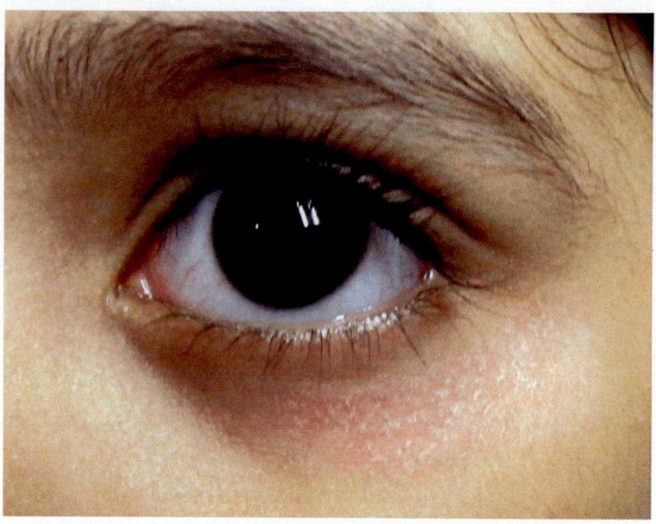

Fig. 3.28: Early eczema around eyes, pigmentation and thinning of lateral eyebrows

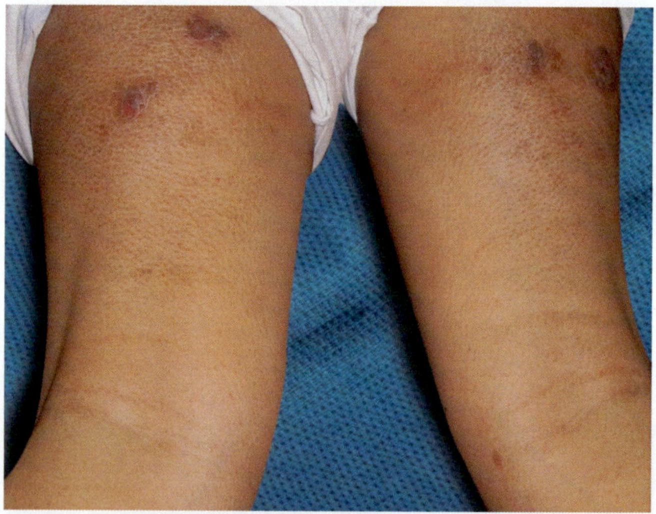

Fig. 3.29: Eczema on posterior aspect of thighs

with UV exposure and polymorphous light eruption like lesions are seen in approximately 3% of patients with adult AD.[5]

Senile AD—senile AD is seen in age above 60 years, characterized by xerosis, lichenified flexural lesions usually are not present (Figs 3.38 and 3.39).

Natural History and Prognosis

Atopic dermatitis is a chronic and chronically relapsing disease with spontaneous improvement in childhood AD as

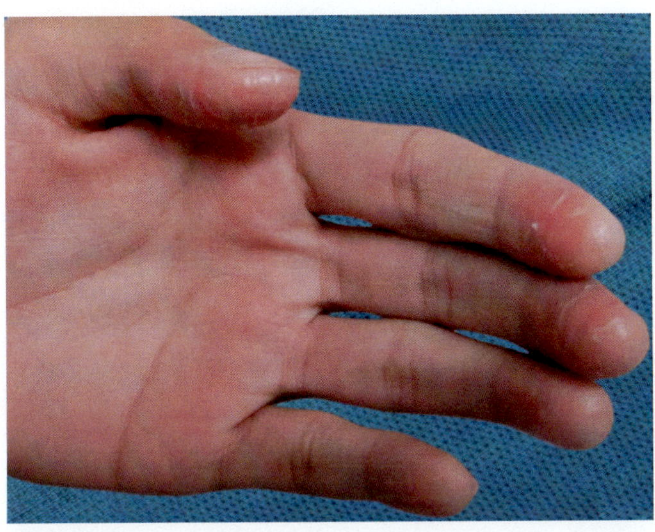

Fig. 3.30: Hand eczema

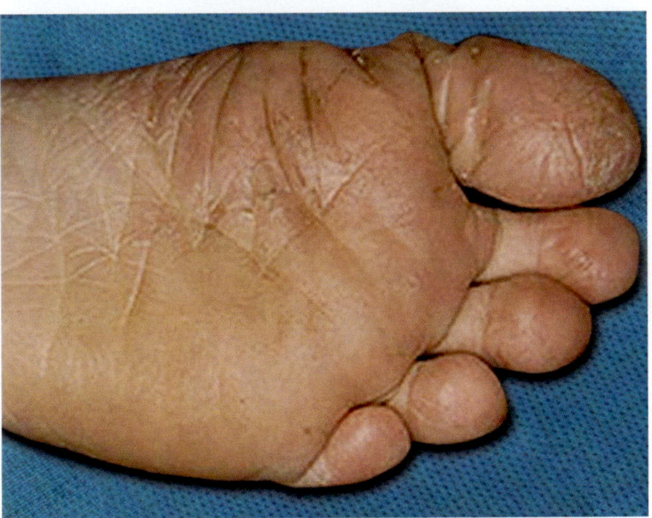

Fig. 3.31: Scaling of soles

age advances and some relapse during adolescence. Around 60% clearance is reported by the age of 10–20 years.[14] Though it is difficult to predict prognosis in an individual case, children having early onset, severe disease, asthma, hay fever and family history of AD have persistent disease. Raised IgE antibodies to foods and inhalant antigens indicate poor prognosis. Adults with involvement of head and neck are likely to have prolonged disease.[15] Atopic children are at risk of having occupational irritant hand dermatitis in adulthood.[16]

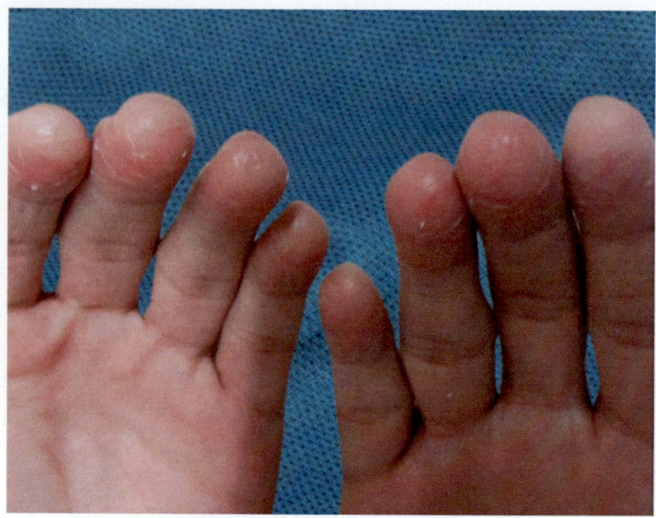

Fig. 3.32: Finger involvement

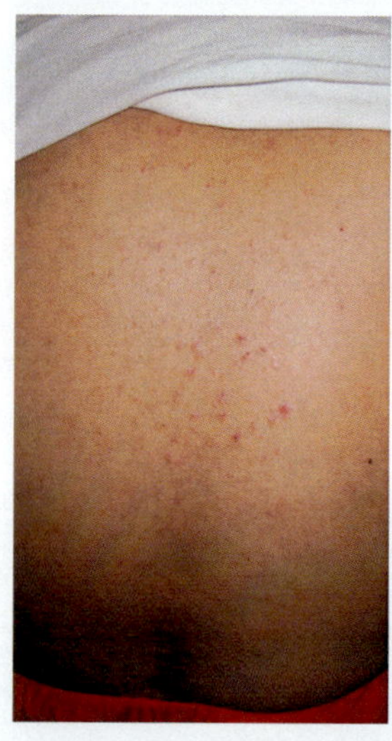

Fig. 3.33: Generalized papular rash

Associated Features and Complications

Periocular and Ocular Signs

Dennie–Morgan lines (infraorbital skin folds) are seen commonly in 50–60% patients of AD, but it is not specific for AD (Fig. 3.39).

'**Atopic shiners**' refers to periorbital brown to gray pigmentation.

'**Hertoghe's sign**' (thinning or absence of lateral eyebrows) may also be present. This sign was originally described in hypothyroidism (Fig. 3.40).

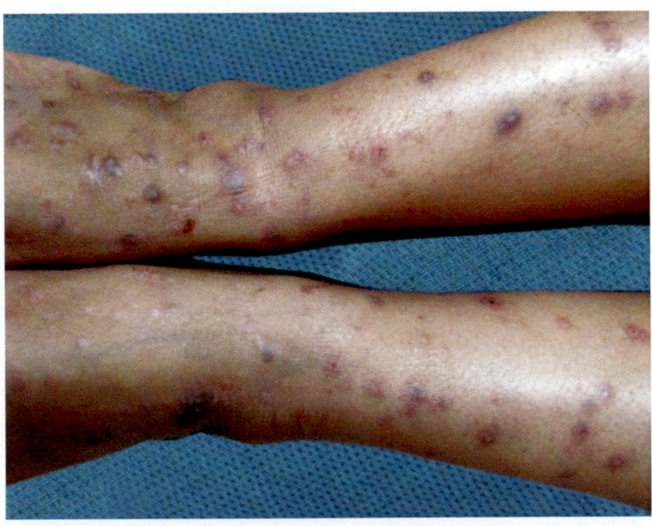

Fig. 3.34: Prurigo-like lesions

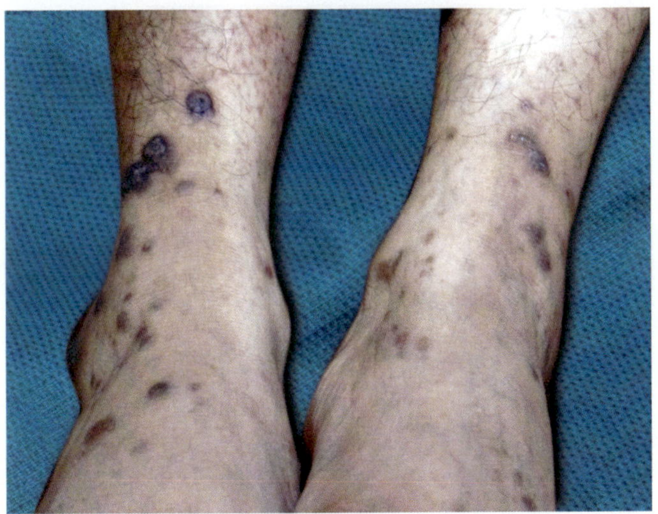

Fig. 3.35: Nodular prurigo-like lesions

Specific Ocular Signs

Conjunctival irritation syndrome is commonly present.

Keratoconus or conical cornea occurs due to degenerative change in cornea which is forced outwards by intraocular pressure resulting in visual disturbances, may occur in association with AD.

Cataracts—cataracts are seen in up to 10% of severe cases of adult and adolescent AD, peak is between 15 and 25 years of age but it may develop from childhood to 30 years of age. Usually they are bilateral, anterior or posterior subcapsular.

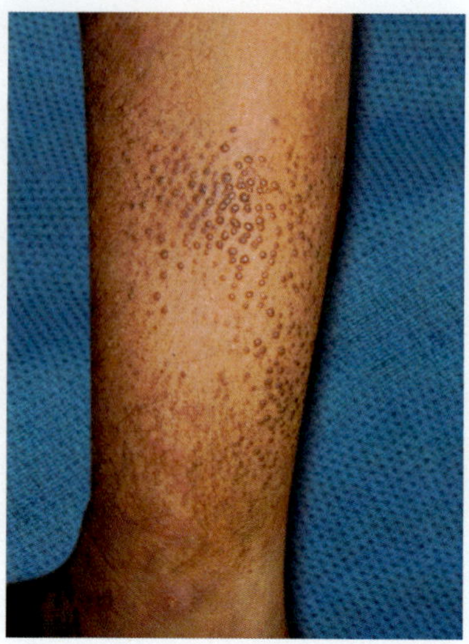

Fig. 3.36: Dark lichenoid lesions

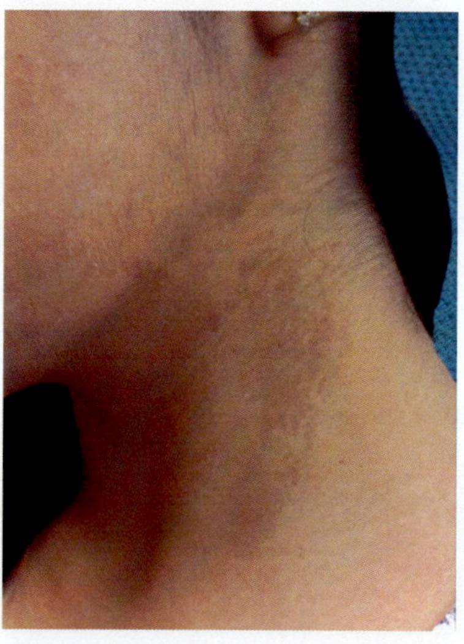

Fig. 3.37: Rash in photosensitive areas

Posterior subcapsular cataracts in AD are indistinguishable from steroid-induced cataracts.

Retinal detachment is also been reported.

Other manifestations associated with AD:

Cutaneous signs—

Prominent nasal crease

'**Dirty-neck appearance** refers to rippled hyperpigmentation of anterior and lateral neck.

Keratosis pilaris seen as horny keratotic papules on upper arms, legs, cheeks, buttocks.

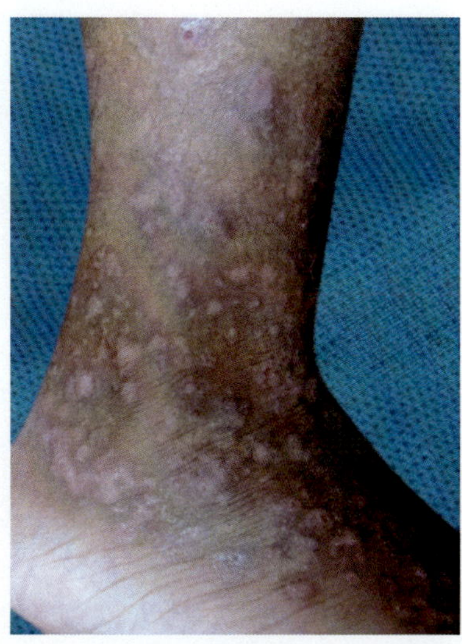

Fig. 3.38: Xerosis and lichenified eczema in adult atopics

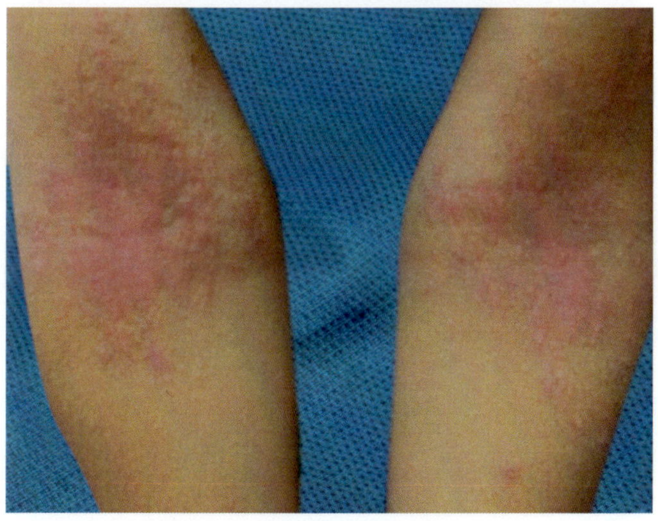

Fig. 3.39: lichenified flexural lesions in adult

Postauricular and infra-auricular involvement leading to ulcerations and fissuring

Fine papular eruptions with dry skin (Fig. 3.41)

Postinflammatory hyper- and hypopigmentation after scratching especially darker Indian skin types (Fig. 3.42)

Prurigo mitis or papular urticarial and prurigo nodularis— sometimes dry thick papulonodules are seen which are easily excoriated, are seen all over body especially hands and feet in easily accessible areas (Fig. 3.43).[2]

Discrete papular lesions around umbilicus (Fig. 3.44)

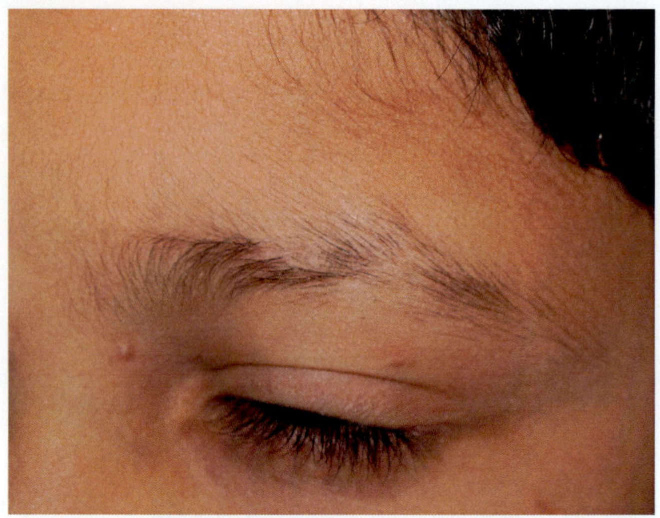

Fig. 3.40: Hertoghe's sign-thinning of lateral side of eyebrows

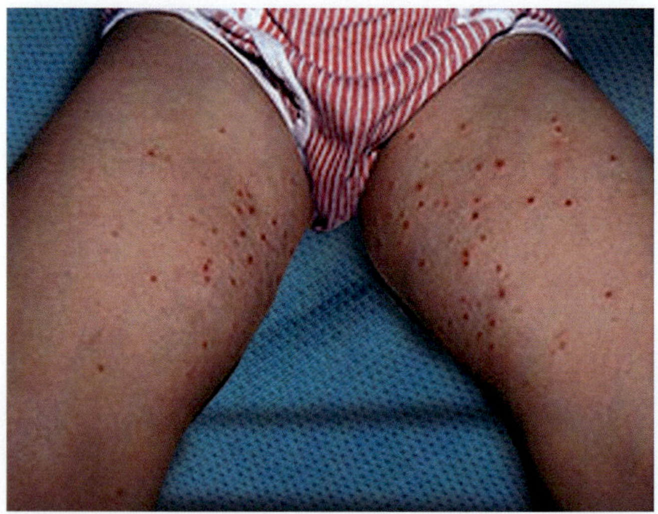

Fig. 3.41: Papular eruptions

Bilateral involvement of thighs and buttocks, so called 'school chair sign' (Fig. 3.45)

Papular and follicular lesions may be sometimes associated (Fig. 3.46).

Dry skin or xerosis characterized by fine scaling and roughness on palpation is seen in all three stages of AD. It is due to increased transepidermal water loss through abnormal stratum corneum and defective ceramide synthesis (Fig. 3.47).[2]

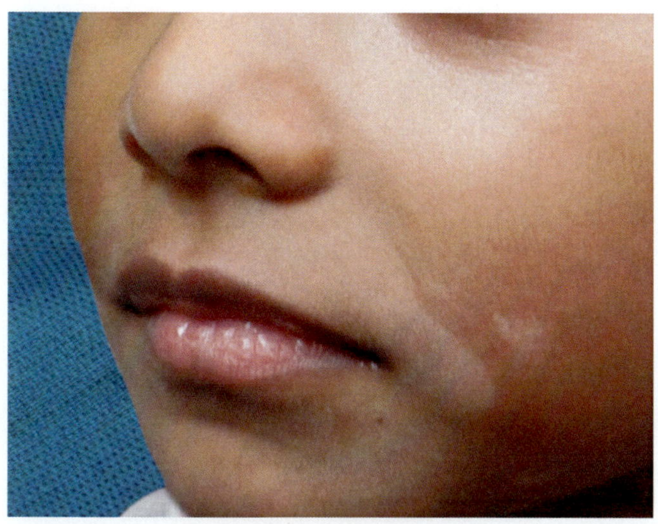

Fig. 3.42: Postinflammatory pigmentary changes after scratching

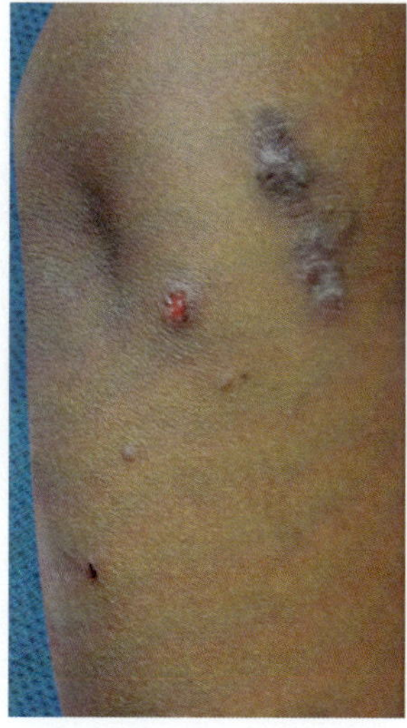

Fig. 3.43: Prurigo mitis or papular urticaria lesion

Palmar hyperlinearity may also be present in AD *supposed to be associated with filaggrin mutation and asthma* (Figs 3.48 to 3.50).

Pityriasis alba seen as ill-defined hypopigmented scaly patches on cheeks and upper arms in children and adolescence (Figs 3.51 and 3.52).

Cheilitis and perioral dermatitis also called as lip licker's dermatitis (Figs 3.53 and 3.54).

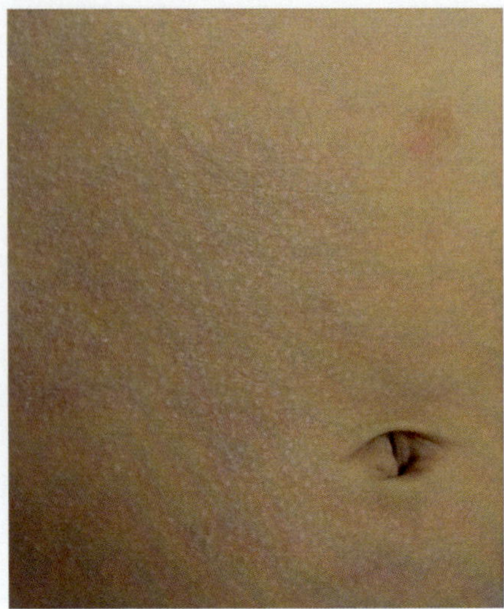

Fig. 3.44: Discrete papular lesions aroud umbilicus

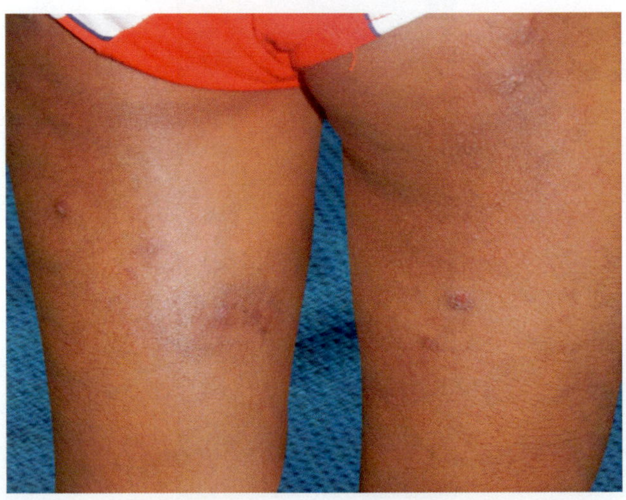

Fig. 3.45: School chair sign—bilateral lesions on thighs or buttocks

Juvenile plantar dermatosis is glazed erythema, scaling and fissuring on the balls of feet and plantar surface of toes in atopic children seen more commonly in winter (Fig. 3.55).

Atopic hand eczema involves dorsum of hands and volar surface of wrists, seen in atopic individuals with frequent exposure to water and irritants. 60% of adult patients with AD are affected with hand eczema (Fig. 3.56).

Discoid eczema (Figs 3.57 and 3.58) usually seen in young adolescents on extensor aspect on extremities, seen as coin-shaped subacute eczematous patch with excoriations.

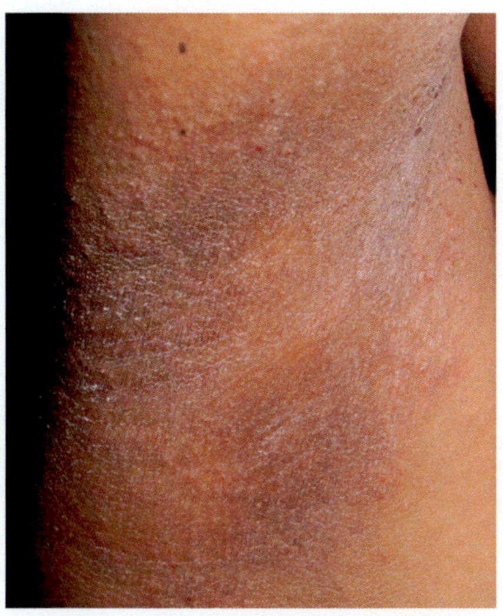

Fig. 3.46: Follicular papular lesions

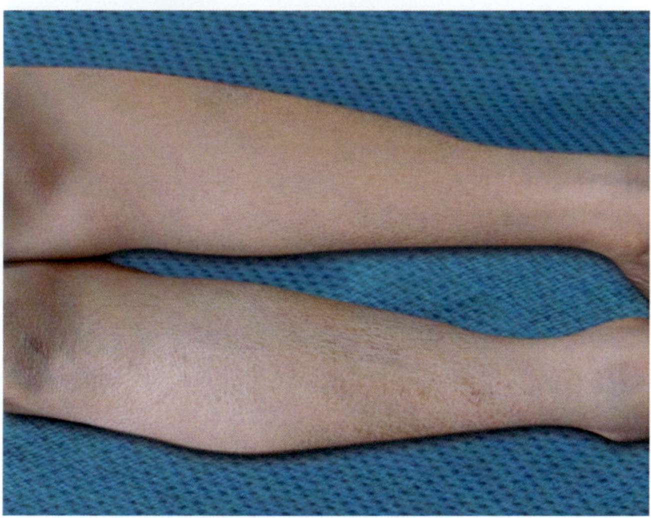

Fig. 3.47: Dry xerotic skin

Dyshidrotic eczema (Fig. 3.59) itchy vesiculation of palms and soles and at lateral margins of fingers and toes are frequent association of atopic eczema.

Nipple eczema may be an association with atopic eczema in young girls and lactating mothers also seen in boys occasionally especially those who take part in strenuous sports.

Alopecia areata is more common in patients with AD (Figs 3.60 and 3.61).

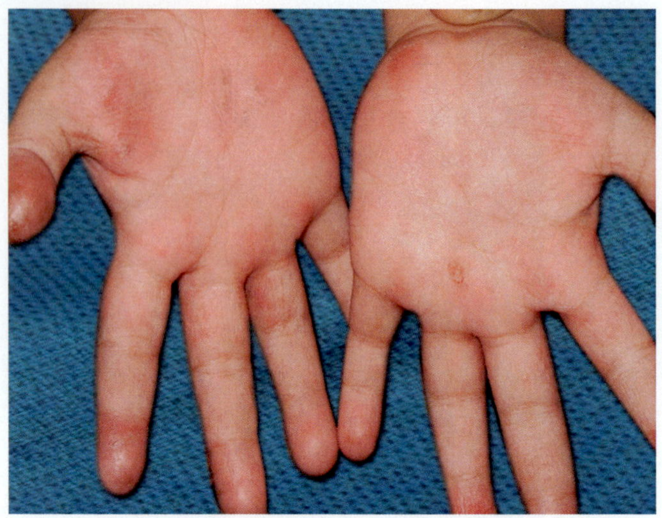

Fig. 3.48: Palmoplantar hyperlinearity and shiny palms

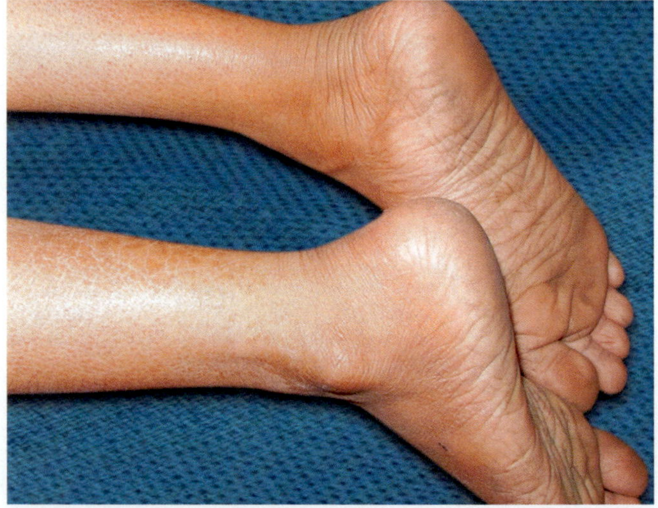

Fig. 3.49: Palmoplantar hyperlinearity and ichthyosis

Vascular Signs

Headlight sign—periorbital, perinasal, perioral pallor.

White dermatographism—blanching of the skin at the site of stroking with blunt instrument.

Urticarias (Figs 3.62 and 3.63) especially contact urticarias are commonly seen especially in food handlers and slaughterhouse workers, in healthcare providers due to sensitivity to latex protein.[2]

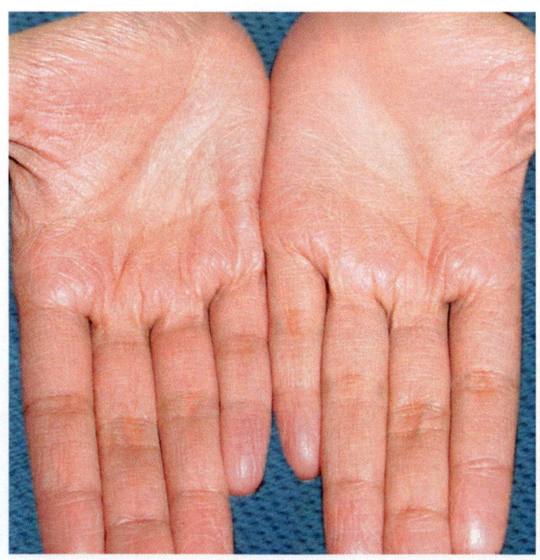

Fig. 3.50: Palmoplantar hyperlinearity and shiny palms

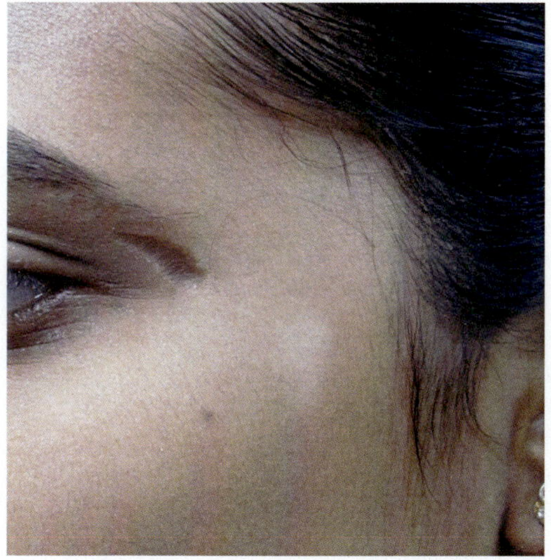

Fig. 3.51: Pityriasis alba

Associated Diseases

Other manifestations of atopy like allergic rhinitis and asthma, 30–50% of atopic patients. Atopic dermatitis is risk factor for future development of allergic airway disease, due to percutaneous sensitization to protein antigen.

Allergic Contact Dermatitis

Patients with AD may develop allergic contact dermatitis to topical medications including antibiotics and corticosteroids.

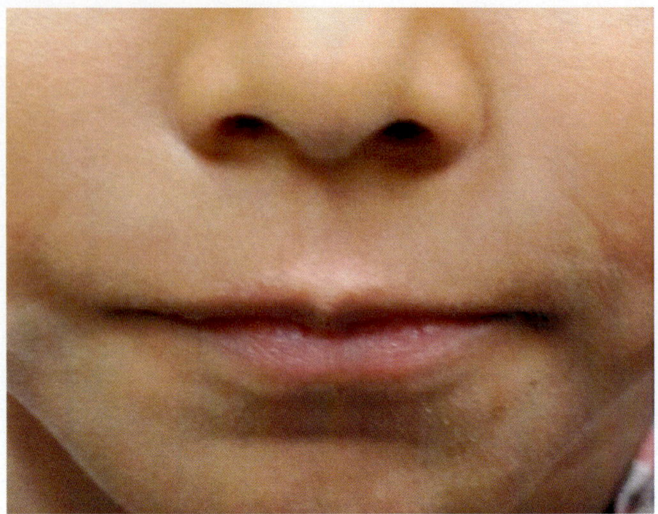

Fig. 3.52: Pityriasis alba

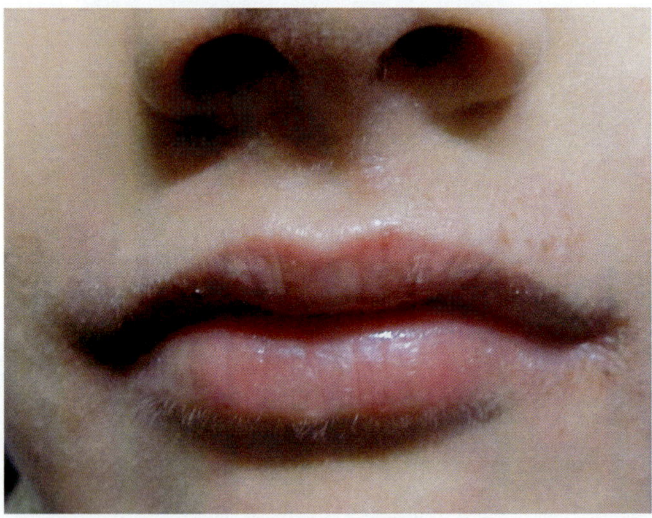

Fig. 3.53: Cheilitis

In a study done by AD. Sharma, 23% of atopic patients had positive patch test and neomycin was found to be the most common allergen (Fig. 3.64).[7]

Lip-lick Cheilitis

Lip-lick cheilitis or perioral eczema is seen as eczematous lesions around mouth in children with atopic dermatitis. It may also be seen with food allergy, toothpaste sensitization.

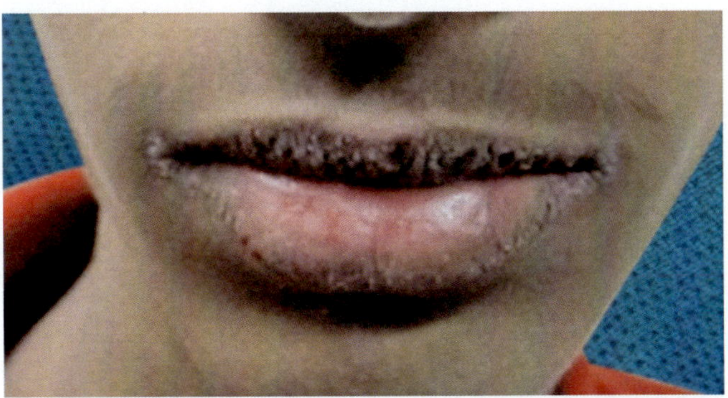

Fig. 3.54: Perioral lesions—lip-licking dermatitis

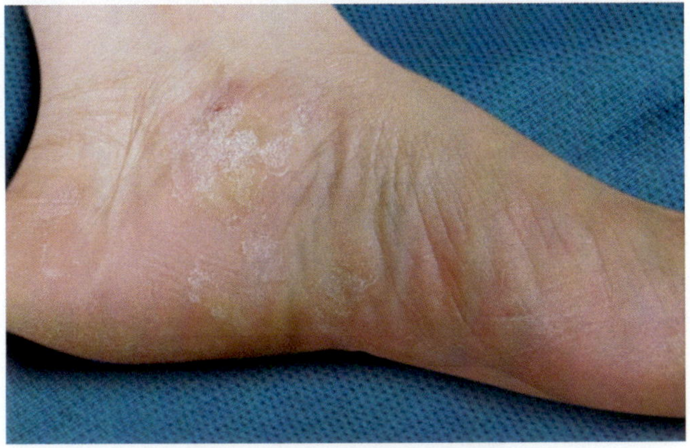

Fig. 3.55: Juvenile plantar dermatitis

Drug sensitivity—IgE-mediated drug reactions of anaphylactic type are commonly seen in atopic patients, anaphylactic reactions to injected antigens, topically applied drugs have been reported.

Food allergy—food hypersensitivity affects 10–30% of infants and children.[13] Most common causative allergens are eggs, milk, peanuts, soy and wheat. Food allergy may cause abdominal symptoms in atopic patients.

Complications

1. Secondary infections

Bacterial infections—secondary bacterial infections are commonly found in patients of AD. *Staphylococcus aureus* and streptococci are causative agents commonly. *Staphylococcus aureus* is found in lesions and normal skin of atopic

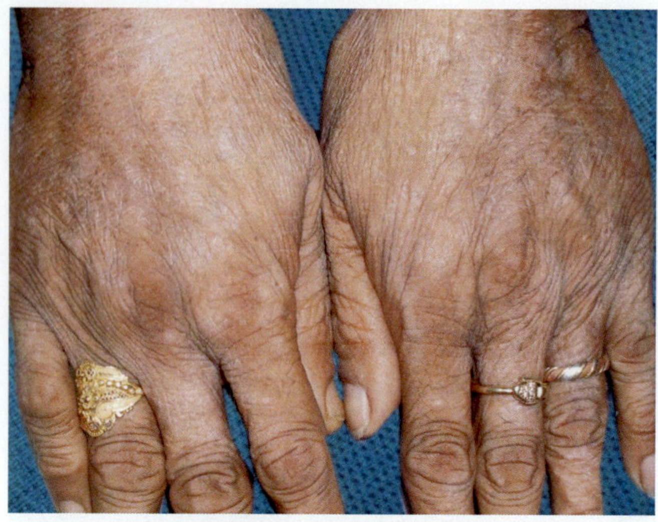

Fig. 3.56: Hand eczema in atopic workers

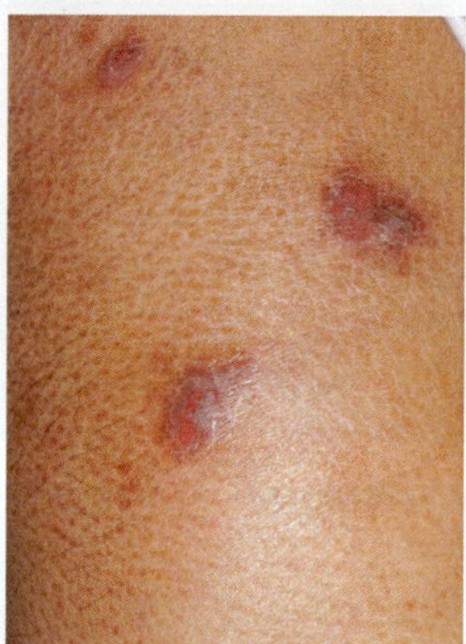

Fig. 3.57: Discoid eczema

individuals. *Staphylococcus aureus* is related to pathogenesis of AD and more severe the AD higher is the rate of colonization with *Staphylococcus aureus*.[8] The presence of exotoxins and other substances from *S. aureus* may act as allergens or, more importantly, as superantigens. Presence of pathogenic staphylococcus in normal skin in atopic individuals result in weeping and crusting of lesions, retroauricular, infra-auricular, perinasal fissures, folliculitis and lymphadenopathy (Fig 3.65). Flares in AD are associated with secondary infections. Treatment with topical steroids results in reduction of pathogenic bacteria on the surface without using antibiotics. Reduction of nasal carriage and treating *Staphylococcus aureus*

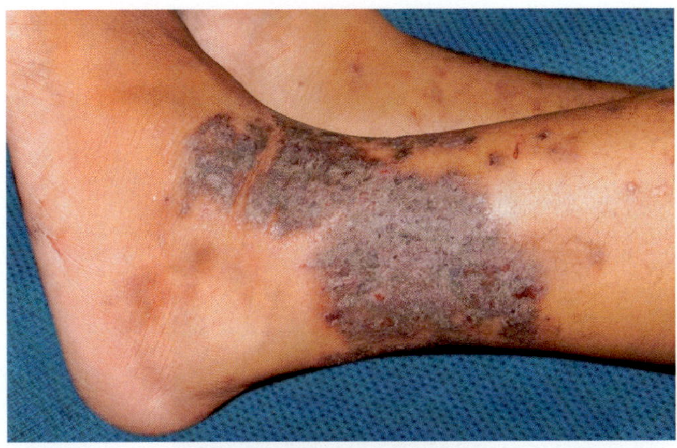

Fig. 3.58: Discoid eczema

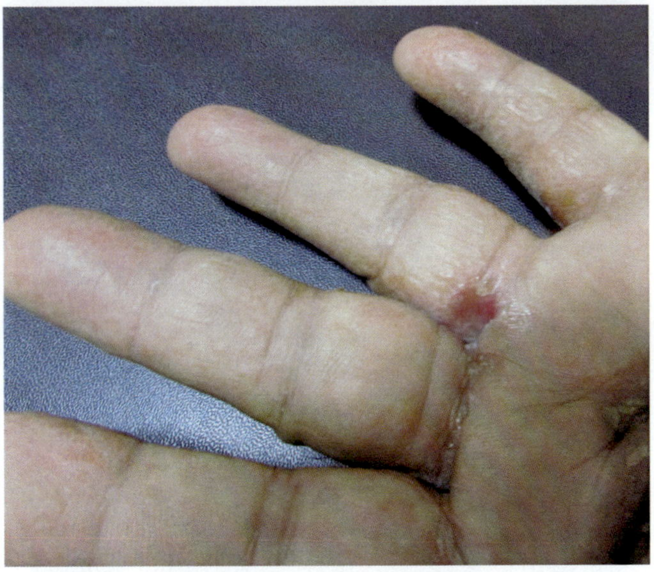

Fig. 3.59: Dyshidrotic eczema

carrier in family is important in controlling infection triggered frequent flares of AD.[5]

Viral infections—atopic dermatitis patients are susceptible to infections with herpes simplex virus. Generalized herpes simplex infection (**Eczema Herpeticum**) occurs mostly with HSV1 but cases with HSV2 have also been described.[9] A monomorphic eruption of dome-shaped blisters, erosions and pustules in eczematous skin with severe systemic illness gives

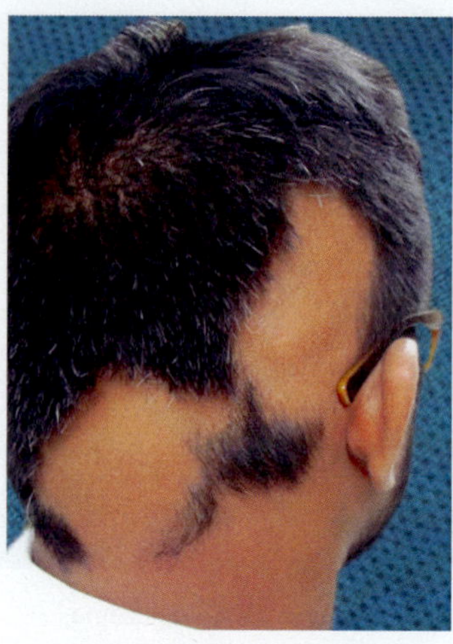

Fig. 3.60: Alopecia areata frequent association with atopic eczema

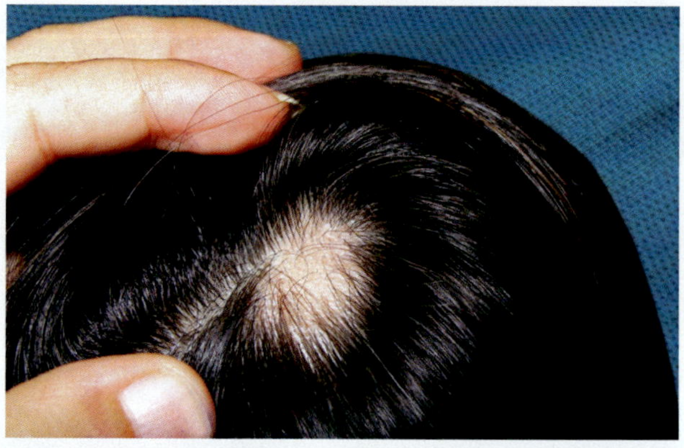

Fig. 3.61: Alopecia areata frequent association with atopic eczema

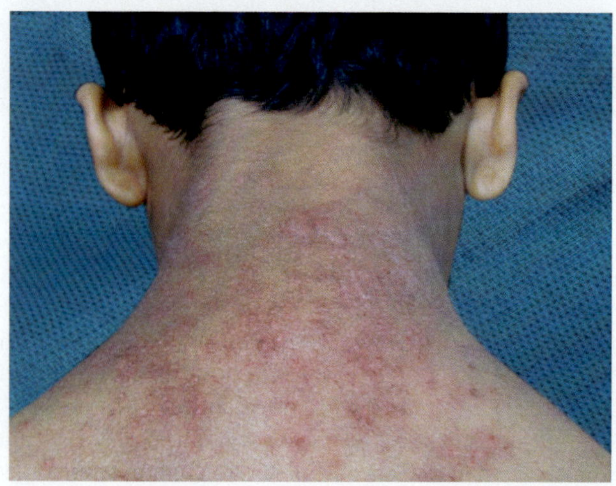

Fig. 3.62: Urticaria and eczema

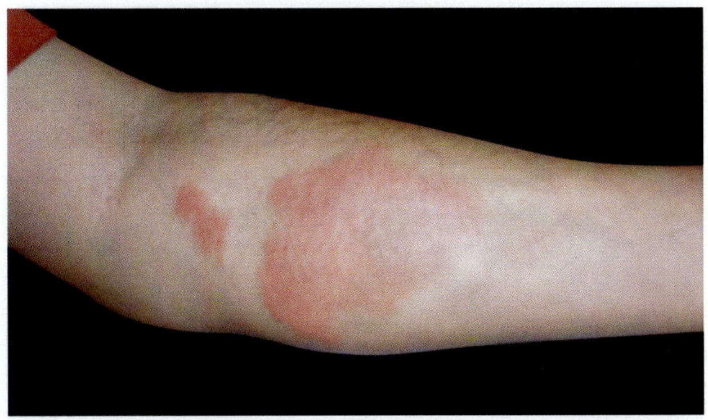

Fig. 3.63: Urticaria

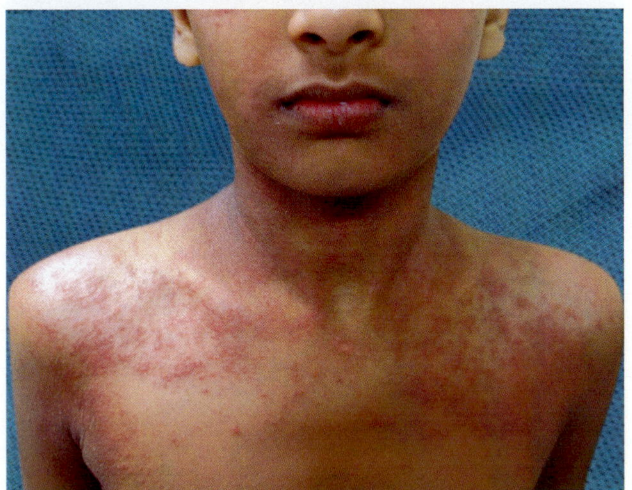

Fig. 3.64: Allergic contact dermatitis

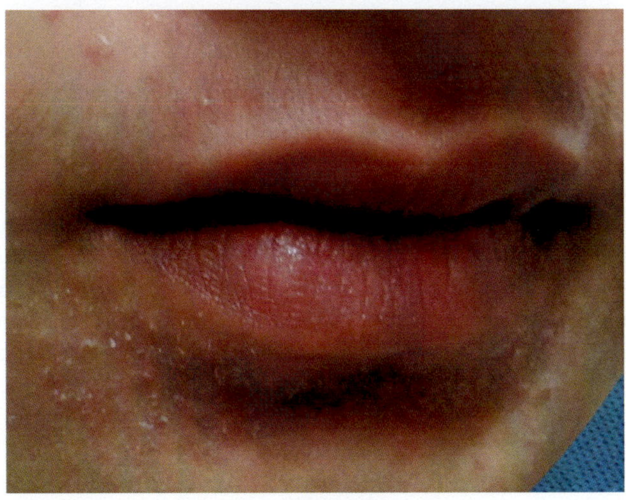

Fig. 3.65: Perioral dermatitis

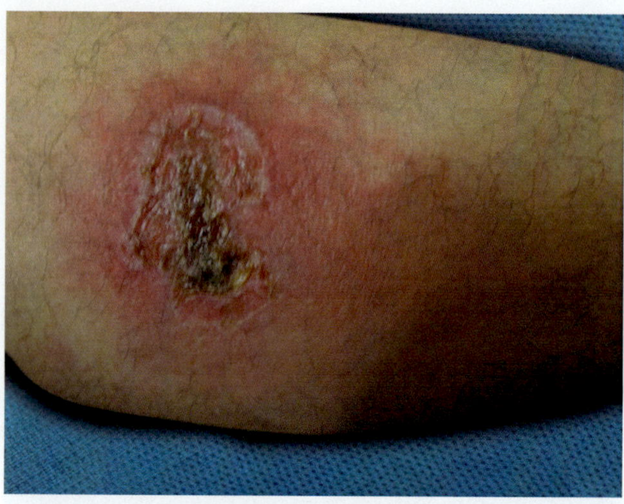

Fig. 3.66: Pyoderma

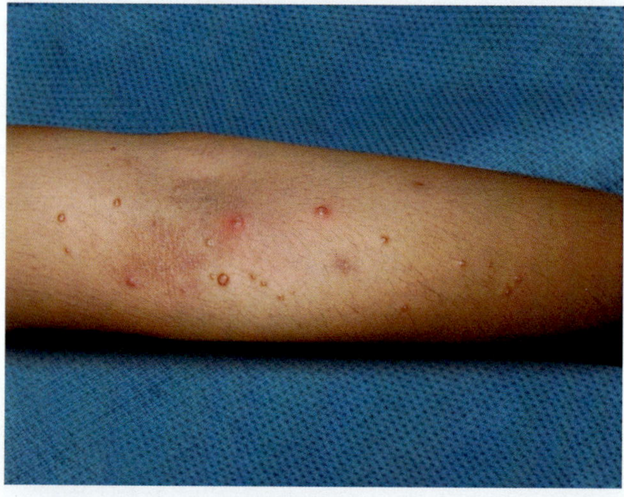

Fig. 3.67: Molluscum contagiosum in atopic individuals

the clue to clinical diagnosis (Fig 3.66). It can be confirmed by Tzanck test, viral culture, polymerase chain reaction, immunofluorescence, electron microscopy with negative staining or serology.Intravenous acyclovir is the treatment of choice, newer oral antiviral drugs are also effective.[10] **Eczema vaccinatum** is widespread vaccinia infection in atopic individuals, it is rare but life threatening. Smallpox vaccination is contraindicated in patients with atopic diathesis even when dermatitis is in remission. Widespread and fatal vaccinia occurs in patients with atopic diathesis.

Widespread molluscum contagiosum (Fig 3.67) is more common in atopic children. Viral infection with papilloma virus early results, leading and multiple warts (Fig 3.68).

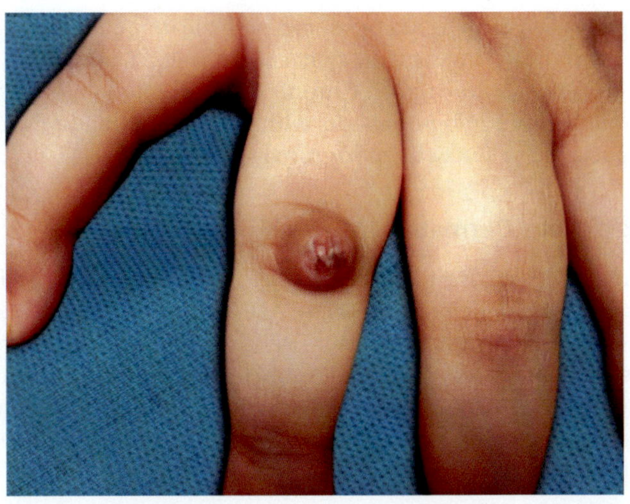

Fig. 3.68: Wart in atopic individuals

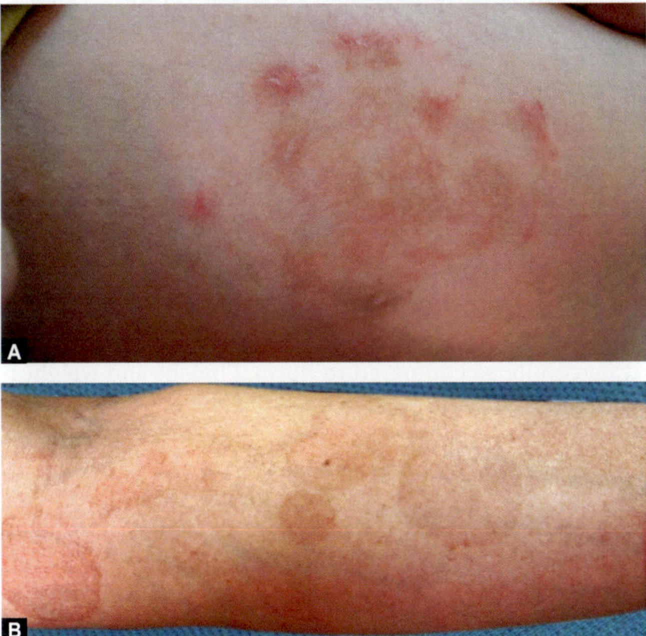

Figs 3.69A and B: Fungal infections in atopic individuals—Incognito with steroid applications

Fungal Infections (Figs 3.69A and B)

The yeasts *Malassezia* and *Candida* may aggravate AD due to an allergic reaction. *Malassezia* species are members of the normal human cutaneous flora, and a defect in the skin barrier may facilitate the contact of these yeasts with the immune system. Candida yeasts are members of the normal flora of mucous membranes, and the major contact with the immune system is through the gastrointestinal tract and, in women, it may occur even through the vagina. Chronic dermatophyte infections are more common in patients with AD, and dermatophytes, especially *Trichophyton rubrum*, may act as allergens.[11]

Exfoliative Dermatitis

Exfoliative dermatitis—exfoliative dermatitis develops in patients with moderate to severe AD, it can occur at any age. In recent onset erythroderma well-established preexisting lesions of AD are present. Intense pruritus, secondary excoriations, prurigo-like lesions, lichenification and atrophy due to topical corticosteroid use is frequently found. Increased serum IgE and eosinophilia is present.

Psychosocial Aspects

Atopic dermatitis affects patients as well as their families due to intense pruritus and chronically relapsing nature. Itching is severe enough to disturb sleep of patients. In children it results in irritability, behavioral difficulties and poor scholastic performance.

Growth Delay

Atopic dermatitis is associated with growth retardation. In an Indian study by Dhar et al. 42% of the AD children had weight below 3rd percentile and 34% atopic children had height below 3rd percentile as compared to normal height and weight in controls.[12]

REFERENCES

1. Simpson EL. Atopic dermatitis: a review of topical treatment options. Curr Med Respopin. 2010;26(3):633-40
2. Friedmann PS, Arden-Jones MR, Holden CA. Atopic Dermatitis. Wiley-Blackwell; 2010.24.19p.
3. Hanifin JM, Rajka G. Diagnostic features of atopic dermatitis. Acta Derm Venerol (Stockh). 1980;92:42-7.
4. Weinberg EG. The Atopic march. Current allergy and clinical immunology. 2005;18(1):4-5.
5. James W, Berger T, Elston D. Atopic dermatitis, eczema and non-infectious, immunodeficiency disorders. Andrew's Diseases of the skin; 11th edn. Elsevier; 2011. PP63-6.
6. Langan S, Williaams C. Clinical features and Diagnostic criteria of Atopic Dermatitis. In: Irvin A, Hoeger P, Yan A (Eds). Harper's Textbook of Paediatric Dermatology; 3rd edn. vol. Wiley-Blackwell; 2011.28.1-19p.

7. Sharma AD. Allergic contact dermatitis in patients with atopic dermatitis: A clinical study. Indian J Dermatol Venereol Leprol. 2005;71:96-8.

8. Gong JQ1, Lin L, Lin T, Hao F, Zeng FQ, Bi ZG, et al. Skin colonization by *Staphylococcus aureus* in patients with eczema and atopic dermatitis and relevant combined topical therapy: a double-blind multicentre randomized controlled trial. Br J Dermatol. 2006;155(4):680-7.

9. David TJ, Longson M. Herpes simplex infections in atopic eczema. Arch Dis child. 1985;60:338-43.

10. Rerinck HC, Kamann S, Wollenberg A. Eczema herpeticum: Pathogenesis and therapy. Hautarzt. 2006;57(7):586-91.

11. Jan Faergemann. Atopic Dermatitis and Fungi. Clin Microbiol Rev. 2002;15(4):545-63.

12. Dhar S, Banerjee R. Atopic dermatitis in infants and children in India. Indian J Dermatol Venereol Leprol. 2010;76:504-13.

13. Bieber T, Bussmann C. Atopic dermatitis. Bolognia J, Jorrings J, Schaffer J (Eds). Dermatology. 3rd edn, vol 1. Elsevier; 2012. p.213.

14. Rajka G. Essential Aspects of Atopic Dermatitis. Berlin: Springer-Verlag; 1989.

15. Williams HC, Wüthrich B. The natural history of atopic dermatitis. In: Williams HC (Ed). Atopic Dermatitis: The Epidemiology, Causes, and Prevention of Atopic Eczema. Cambridge: Cambridge University Press; 2000.pp. 41-59.

16. Illi S, von Mutius E, Lau S, et al. The natural course of atopic dermatitis from birth to age 7 years and the association with asthma. J Allergy Clin Immunol 2004;113:925-31.

Diagnosis and Differential Diagnosis

Shylaja Somshwar, Satish Udare

DIAGNOSIS

Diagnosis of atopic dermatitis (AD) is based on a constellation of signs and symptoms as there are no laboratory "gold standard" for the diagnosis of AD. The definitive diagnosis of AD requires the presence of all three of the following features: Pruritus, typical morphology and distribution, and chronic and chronically relapsing course. In majority of the cases, the diagnosis is quite easily made in routine dermatologist office with the help of signs and symptoms, history, morphology and distribution of skin lesions and associated clinical signs. However, it may prove difficult in certain situations, e.g. in early stage of the disease, during remission and when the morphology of the skin lesions have been modified by treatment.

As it shows variable clinical features and because of lack of an objective diagnostic test for its diagnosis, it poses difficulties in diagnosis and management. In this regard it was Hanifin and Rajka who came up with the diagnostic criteria during the International Symposium on Atopic Dermatitis, that was organized in Oslo, 7–9 June 1979 and published in 1980[1] based on clinical features which was followed for 14 long years (Table 4.1).

The presence of 3 major and 3 minor criteria are necessary for the diagnosis.

Though it was extensively followed, certain difficulties were encountered in following the Hanifin and Rajka criteria:

a. It consists of a long list of 27 features and thus, is time consuming. For clinical studies these criteria were found to be useful but they were found unsuitable for population-based studies[2,3]

b. Only two validation studies of the complete Hanifin and Rajka criteria have been published in spite of the criteria being quoted in a number of scientific studies.

To overcome these problems, the UK diagnostic criteria (Table 4.2) was introduced in 1994 by Williams et al. with the aim of developing a minimum list of reliable discriminators.[4]

Table 4.1: Hanifin and Rajka's criteria for the diagnosis of atopic dermatitis[1]

Major/basic features
- Pruritus
- Typical morphology and distribution: Flexural lichenification or linearity in adults, facial and extensor involvement in infants and children
- Chronic or chronically relapsing dermatitis
- Personal or family history of atopy [asthma, allergic rhinitis (AR), AD]

Minor or less-characteristic features
- Xerosis
- Ichthyosis/palmar hyperlinearity/keratosis pilaris
- Immediate (type 1) skin test reactivity
- Elevated serum IgE
- Early age at onset
- Tendency towards cutaneous infections (especially *Staphylococcus Aureus* and Herpes simplex)/impaired cell-mediated immunity
- Tendency towards nonspecific hand or foot dermatitis
- Nipple eczema
- Cheilitis
- Recurrent conjunctivitis
- Dennie–Morgan infraorbital folds
- Keratoconus
- Anterior subcapsular cataracts
- Orbital darkening
- Facial pallor/facial erythema
- Pityriasis alba
- Anterior neck folds
- Itch when sweating
- Intolerance to wool or lipid solvents
- Perifollicular accentuation
- Food intolerance
- Course influenced by environmental/emotional factors
- White dermographism/delayed blanch

Table 4.2: UK diagnostic criteria

The UK refinement of the Hanifin and Rajka diagnostic criteria for atopic dermatitis[4]

Must have:

An itchy skin condition (or parental report of scratching or rubbing) in the past 12 months

Plus three or more of the following:

History of involvement of the skin creases (fronts of elbows, behind knees, fronts of ankles, around neck or around eyes)

Personal history of asthma or hay fever (or history of atopic disease in first-degree relative if child aged >4 years)

History of generally dry skin in the past year

Onset before the age of 2 years (not used if child aged <4 years)

Visible flexural dermatitis (including dermatitis affecting cheeks or forehead and outer areas of limbs in children aged <4 years)

The original UK criteria cannot be applied to very young children, although revisions to include infants have since been proposed.

It consists of one mandatory and five major criteria, and are more practical for daily practice.

These criteria have been extensively validated in both hospital and epidemiological settings.[5]

A consensus conference was held by the American Academy of Dermatology in January 2001 to address the dermatological issues related to AD in children and adolescents and came up with the clinical criteria (Table 4.3).[6]

The above 3 criteria have specificity at or above 90%, but have much lower sensitivities (40–100%). Therefore, they are useful for enrolling patients in studies and ensuring that they have AD, but are not so useful in diagnosing a specific patient with AD.[7]

In 1998, JD Bos et al. proposed the Millennium criteria where allergen-specific IgE is a mandatory criterion after the better understanding of the pathogenesis of the disease (Table 4.4).[8]

There have been many attempts to define criteria for the diagnosis of AD from across the globe till 2007.[1,4,8-15]

The difficulty of choosing a reliable diagnostic criteria from a pool of them necessitated Brenninkmeijer EE et al. to conduct a systematic review of the same. They undertook a methodological systematic review of 27 published validation studies of various diagnostic criteria for AD. They concluded

---

Table 4.3: Consensus conference on pediatric atopic dermatitis criteria[6]

A. Essential features (must be present)
1. Pruritus
2. Eczema (acute, subacute, chronic)
   a. Typical morphology and age-specific patterns (Patterns include (1) facial, neck, and extensor involvement in infants and children, (2) current or prior flexural lesions in any age group, (3) sparing of groin and axillary regions.)
   b. Chronic or relapsing history

B. Important features (seen in most cases, adding support to the diagnosis)
1. Early age at onset
2. Atopy
   a. Personal and/or family history
   b. IgE reactivity
3. Xerosis

C. Associated features (these clinical associations help to suggest the diagnosis of AD but are too nonspecific to be used for defining or detecting AD for research or epidemiologic studies)
1. Atypical vascular responses (eg, facial pallor, white dermographism, delayed blanch response)
2. Keratosis pilaris/hyperlinear palms/ichthyosis
3. Ocular/periorbital changes
4. Other regional findings (e.g., perioral changes/periauricular lesions)
5. Perifollicular accentuation/lichenification/prurigo lesions

<table>
<tr><td colspan="1">Table 4.4: The millennium criteria for the diagnosis of atopic dermatitis[8]</td></tr>
</table>

1. Mandatory criterion
Presence of allergen-specific IgE:
- Historical, actual, or expected (in very young children)
- In peripheral blood (RAST, ELISA) or in skin (intracutaneous challenge)

2. Principal criteria (2 of 3 present) typical distribution and morphology of eczema lesions: infant, childhood, or adult type
- If distribution is not typical, exclude other entity (dyshidrotic eczema, contact dermatitis, contact urticaria)
- Pruritus
- Chronic or chronically relapsing course

that the UK Working Party's refinement of the Hanifin and Rajka criteria had been the most extensively validated (19 studies), with a sensitivity ranging from 10% to 100% and a specificity from 89 to 99%.[16]

Exclusionary conditions: It should be noted that a diagnosis of AD depends on excluding conditions, such as scabies, seborrheic dermatitis, allergic contact dermatitis, ichthyoses, cutaneous lymphoma, psoriasis, and immune deficiency diseases.

The PRACTALL Program is a common initiative with membership from the European Academy of Allergy and Clinical Immunology (EAACI) and the American Academy of Immunology. The program was called the PRACTALL program (for "practical allergy") and led to the development of a consensus report to guide clinical practice in the diagnosis and treatment of atopic eczema (AE) in children and adults.[17]

LABORATORY STUDIES IN ATOPIC DERMATITIS

- There are no specific tests which will either diagnose the disease, assess severity or give prediction of the course
- These are usually done to additionally prove the diagnosis or establish the differential diagnosis
- These may help in diagnosing immunodeficiencies, secondary infections
- Routine hemogram may show eosinophilia
- Increase in IgE levels may be present in about 80% of individuals with AD
- Skin biopsy though not specific for AD may help in differentiating some other disorders
- Allergy testing such as prick test and blood tests like radioallergosorbent assay (RAST) and patch testing may be useful in certain individuals.

The exposure of AD patients to aeroallergens or food allergens can exacerbate or maintain the disease. Atopy patch tests (APTs) are able to identify these triggering factors and consist of the epicutaneous application of allergens for 48 hours, with an evaluation of the eczematous lesions induced after 48 and 72 hours, according to the reading criteria of the European Task Force on Atopic Dermatitis (ETFAD).[18] It consists of purified allergen preparations in petrolatum, applied in 12-mm diameter Finn chambers mounted on Scanpor tape to non-irritated, non-abraded, or tape-stripped skin of the upper back. The APT is read at 48 and 72 hours according to the test criteria and reading key of the ETFAD for appearance of erythema, and number and distribution pattern of the papules.[19]

REFERENCES

1. Hanifin JM, Rajka G. Diagnostic features of atopic dermatitis. Acta Derm Venereol Suppl (Stockh). 1980;92:44-7.
2. Schultz LF, Hanifin JM. Secular change in the occurrence of atopic dermatitis. Acta Derm Venereol Suppl (Stockh). 1992; 176:7-12.
3. Svensson A, Edman B, Moller H. A diagnostic tool for atopic dermatitis based on clinical criteria. Acta Derm Venereol Suppl (Stockh). 1985;114:33-40.
4. Williams HC, Burney PG, Hay RJ, et al. The UK Working Party's Diagnostic Criteria for Atopic Dermatitis. I. Derivation of a minimum set of discriminators for atopic dermatitis. Br J Dermatol. 1994;131:383-96.
5. Firooz A, Davoudi SM, Farahmand AN, Majdzadeh R, Kashani N, Dowlati Y. Validation of the diagnostic criteria for atopic dermatitis. Arch Dermatol. 1999;135(5):514-6.
6. Eichenfield LF1, Hanifin JM, Luger TA, Stevens SR, Pride HB. Consensus conference on pediatric atopic dermatitis. J Am Acad Dermatol. 2003;49(6):1088-95.
7. James WD, Berger T, Elston D. In Andrew's Diseases of the Skin: Clinical Dermatology. 11th edition. Elsevier Health Sciences; 2011.
8. Bos JD, Van Leent EJ, Sillevis Smitt JH. The millennium criteria for the diagnosis of atopic dermatitis. Exp Dermatol. 1998;7: 132-8.
9. Asher mi, Keil U, Anderson HR, et al. International Study of Asthma and Allergies in childhood (ISAAC): rationale and methods. Eur Respir J. 1995;8:483-91.
10. Diepgen TL, Sauerbrei W, Fartasch M. Development and validation of diagnostic scores in atopic dermatitis incorporating criteria of data quality and practical usefulness. J Clin Epidemiol. 1996;49;1031-8.
11. Johnke H, Vach W, Norberg LA, et al. A comparison between criteria for diagnosing atopic eczema in infants. Br J Dermatol. 2005;153:352-8.

12. Schultz LF, Hanifin JM. Secular change in the occurrence of atopic dermatitis. Acta Derm Venereol Suppl (Stockh). 1992; 176:7-12.
13. Schultz LF, Diepgen T, Svensson A. Clinical criteria in diagnosing atopic dermatitis: the Lillehammer criteria 1994. Acta Derm Venereol Suppl (Stockh). 1996;96:115-9.
14. Kang KF, Tian RM. Criteria for atopic dermatitis in a Chinese population. Acta Derm Venereol Suppl (Stockh). 1989;144:26-7.
15. Tagami H. Japanese Dermatology Association criteria for the diagnosis of atopic dermatitis. J Dermatol. 1995;22:966-7.
16. Brenninkmeijer EE, Schram ME, Leeflang MM, et al. Diagnostic criteria for atopic dermatitis: a systematic review. Br J Dermatol. 2008;158(4):754-65.
17. Wöhrl. Diagnosis and Prevention of atopic eczema. In: Norman RA (ed). Preventive Dermatol. New York: Springer; 2010.137-50.
18. Nosbaum A, Hennino A, Berard F, Nicolas JF. Patch testing in atopic dermatitis patients. Eur J Dermatol. 2010;20:563-6.
19. Kerschenlohr K, Darsow U, Burgdorf WH, Ring J, Wollenberg A. Lessons from atopy patch testing in atopic dermatitis. Curr Allergy Asthma Rep. 2004;4(4):285-9.

DIFFERENTIAL DIAGNOSIS

There are a vast number of diseases which can mimic AD as the condition does not have a classical diagnostic clinical manifestation. Moreover as almost all the features are secondary to pruritus, any generalized itchy dermatosis can imitate AD.

- *Other eczemas*
  - *Allergic/irritant dermatitis (Fig. 4.1)*
    - History plays an important role in distinguishing the two in many cases. Acute onset without prior history of similar complaints may be useful in arriving at the diagnosis though atopic individuals are prone for allergic/irritant dermatitis
    - Maximum lesions at the sites of maximum contact with the irritants/allergens usually on the hands is useful in arriving at the diagnosis
    - Eliminating the suspected cause with treatment of the condition usually cures allergic/irritant dermatitis
    - Patch testing may be helpful in difficult cases.
  - *Seborrheic dermatitis (Fig. 4.2)*
    - In an infant, seborrheic dermatitis is the most common differential diagnosis[1]
    - In early life, cradle cap and diaper area involvement may be commonly seen in a case of seborrheic dermatitis
    - Typical distribution with greasy scales points to the diagnosis of seborrheic dermatitis.
  - *Asteatotic eczema (Fig. 4.3)*
    - Eczematous lesions on the background of xerosis with winter exacerbation is typical of this condition.
  - Id reaction (disseminated eczema)
- *Papulosquamous diseases*
  - *Psoriasis (Figs 4.4 and 4.5)*
    - Though typical distribution of the lesions aid in the diagnosis, when generalized, may pose difficulties
    - Nail changes of psoriasis may be classical
    - Biopsy is usually suggestive of the diagnosis.
  - *Pityriasis rosea (Figs 4.6 and 4.7)*
    - History of mother patch with typical distribution of lesions and a self-limiting course are helpful to diagnose pityriasis rosea
    - Histopathology may help in difficult cases
  - *Pityriasis rubra pilaris (Fig. 4.8)*
    - Typical course of the disease, islands of sparing, follicular hyperkeratosis on an erythematous base, palmoplantar keratoderma are features of pityriasis rubra pilaris

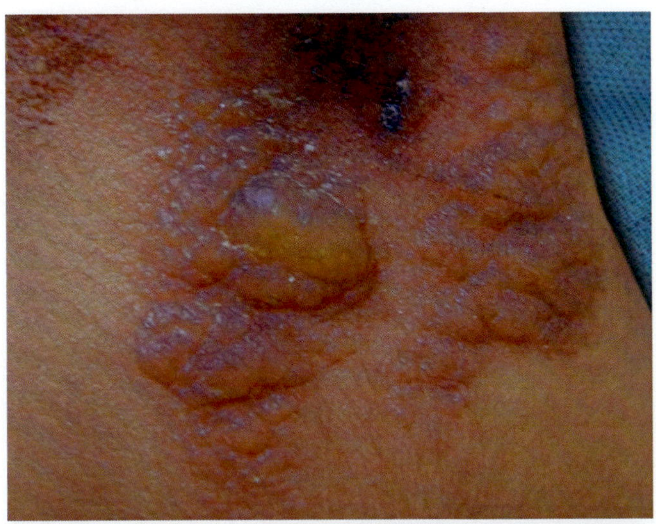

Fig. 4.1: Contact dermatitis

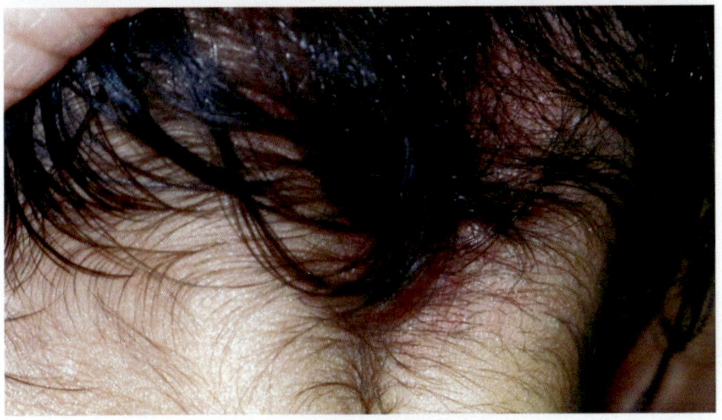

Fig. 4.2: Seborrheic dermatitis

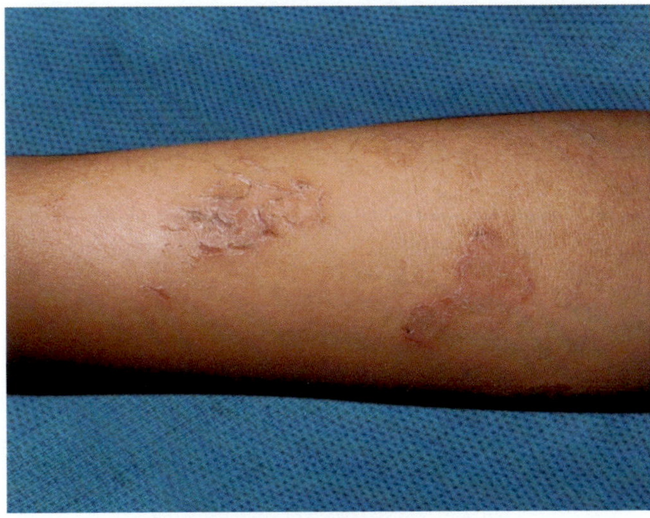

Fig. 4.3: Asteatotic eczema

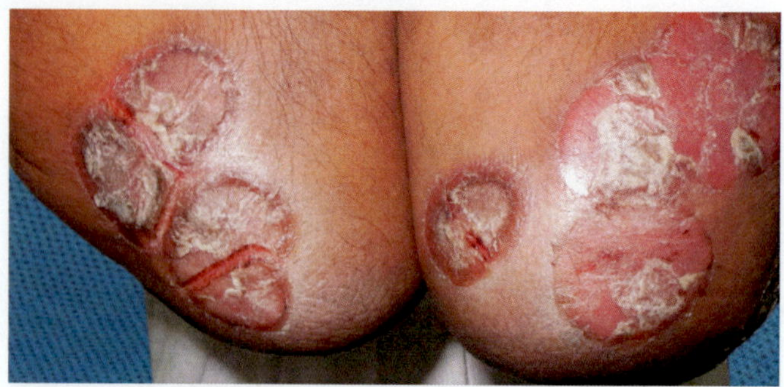

Fig. 4.4: Classic psoriatic plaques on elbows

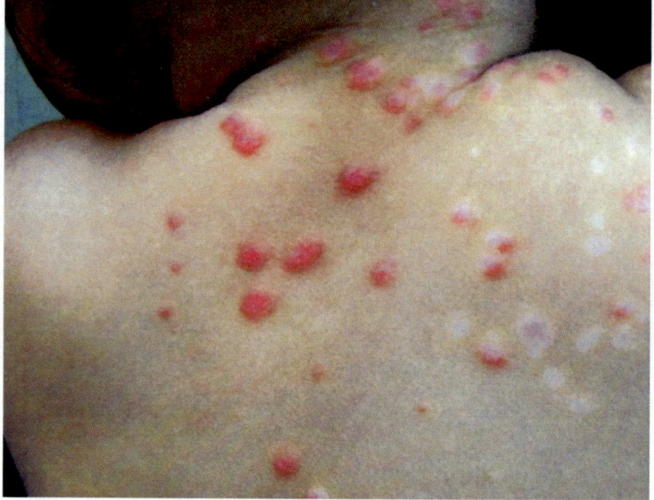

Fig. 4.5: Guttate psoriasis in child after URT (upper respiratory tract infection)

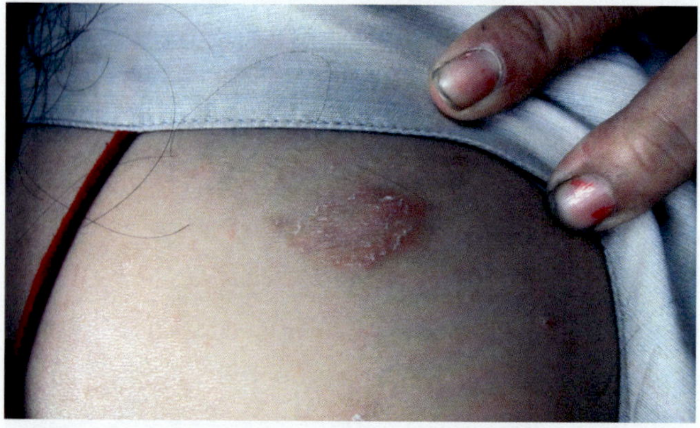

Fig. 4.6: Mother patch of Pityriasis rosea

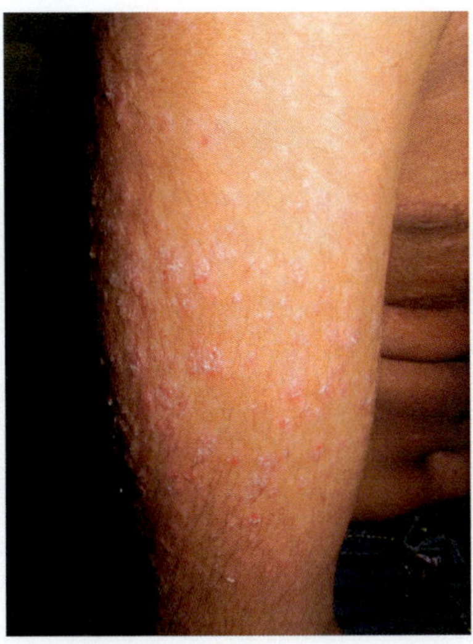

Fig. 4.7: Extensive lesions of Pityriasis rosea

- Lichen planus—extensive widespread lichen planus may pose problem as the disease may be very itchy and lesions may get excoriated, but the classic violaceous hue may help in diagnosis (Figs 4.9 and 4.10)
- Amyloidosis may pose problems of severely itchy papules on hands and feet.
- *Infections and infestations*
  - *Scabies (Fig. 4.11)*
    - Scabies in babies often undergoes eczematization, particularly over the face, quite closely simulating AD[1]
    - Typical distribution of lesions, nocturnal exacerbation and family history of itching if present helps in the diagnosis of scabies
    - Skin scrapings may be positive for mites in scabies.
  - *Viral exanthems (Fig 4.12 and 4.13)*
    - Short course of the disease with a uniformly distributed blanchable erythema are suggestive of this condition.
  - *Extensive dermatophytosis (Fig. 4.14 and 4.15)*
    - Rarely confused with AD. Annular lesions with peripheral scaling is characteristic
    - KOH mount may be positive in fungal infections
    - Atopic individuals are prone for infections.
  - HIV associated dermatitis—many a times there are changes in the skin which may mimic AD. These include dry itchy scaly skin, lichenified lesions, prurigo nodularis like lesions. There may be staphylococcal colonization and infections,

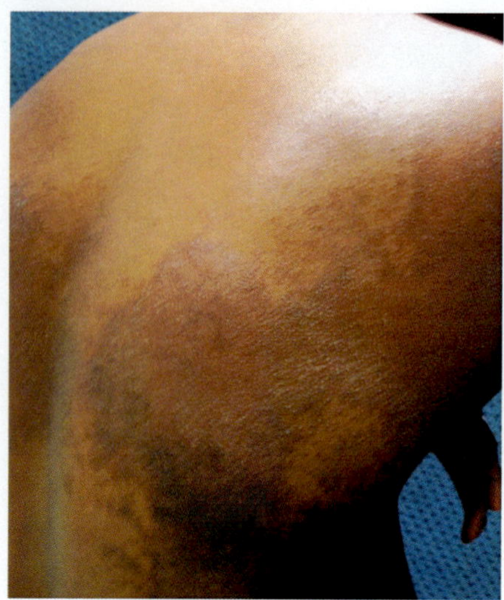

Fig. 4.8: Pityriasis rubra pilaris

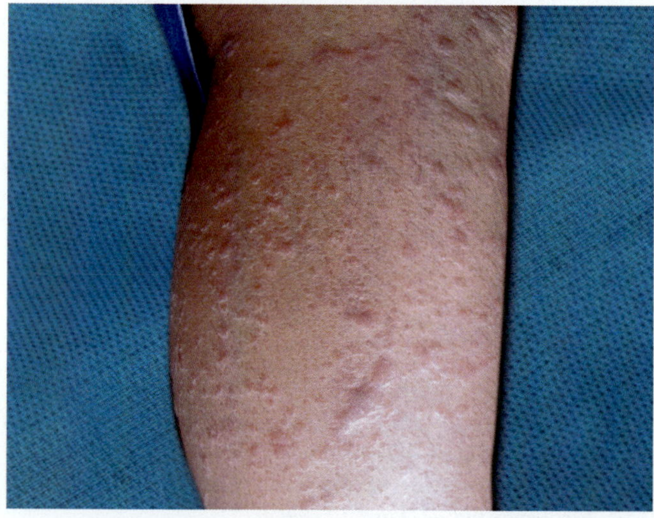

Fig. 4.9: Acute wide-spread lichen planus

folliculitis and similarly there may be increased incidence of fungal and viral infections and infestations. The barrier function may be impaired. There may be increased levels of IgE and eosinophilia in HIV-infected persons leading to the probability that either atopic disease may manifest in HIV-affected individuals or actually increase the severity of the disease.[2]

- *Malignancies*
  - *Cutaneous T cell lymphoma (mycosis fungoides and Sezary syndrome)*

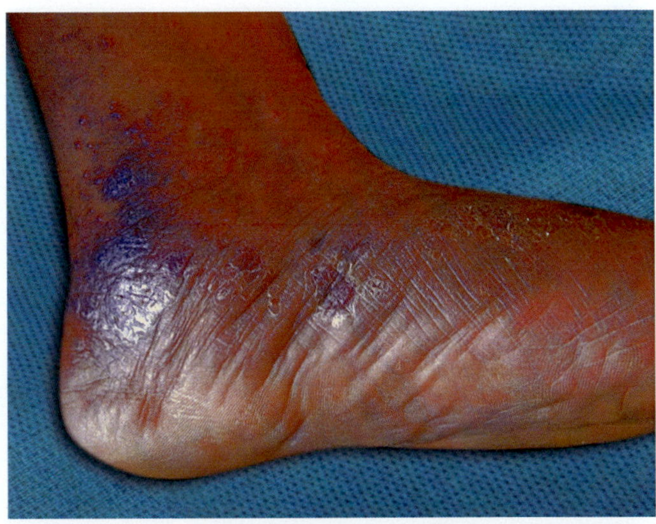

Fig. 4.10: Lichen planus

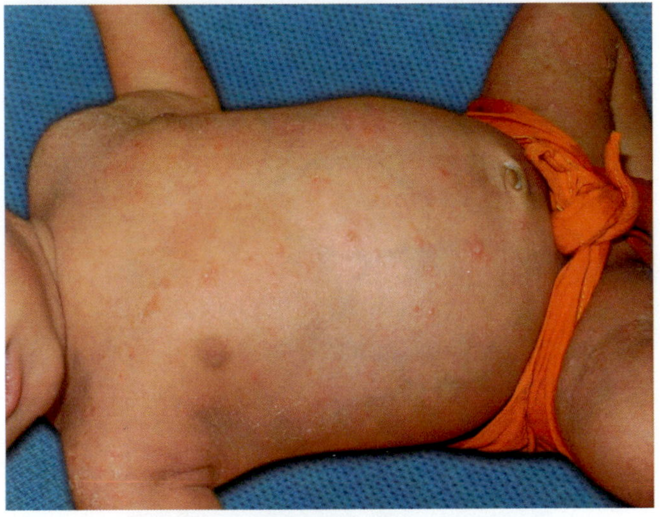

Fig. 4.11: Scabies

- ♦ Suspected in patients presenting with chronic dermatitis poorly responsive to conventional therapy
- ♦ Skin and lymph node biopsies give clue to the diagnosis
- ♦ Histopathological evaluation of multiple sites and immunohistochemistry may help to clinch the diagnosis.
- – *Langerhans cell histiocytosis*

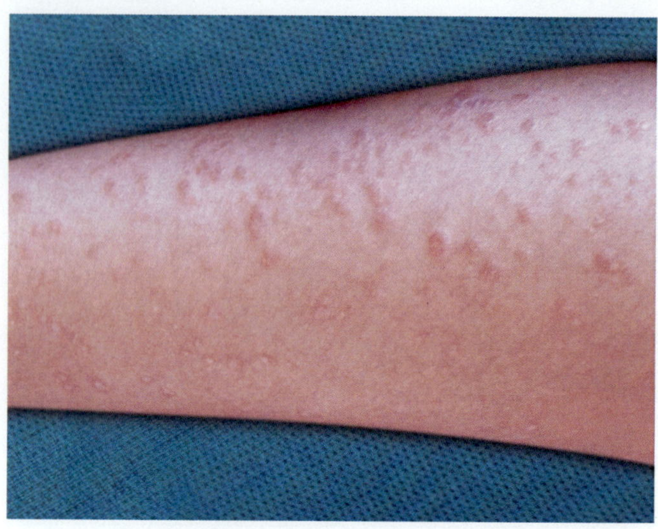

Fig. 4.12: Gianotti–Crosti syndrome

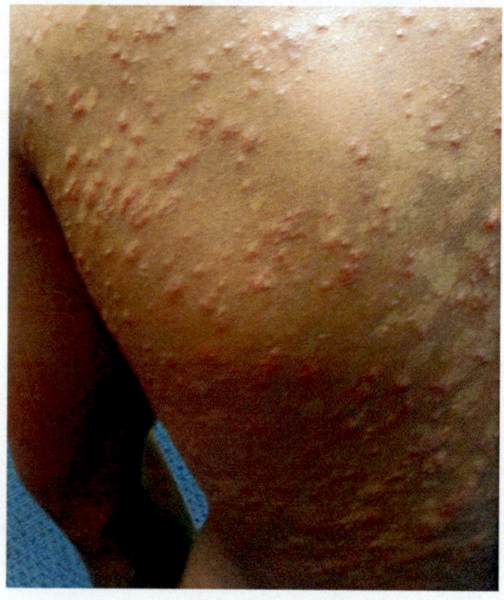

Fig. 4.13: Viral exanthems

- *Immunological deficiencies:* Suspected when infants present with severe eczematous rash with failure to thrive, recurrent infections or petechiae.[2]
  - *Wiskott–Aldrich syndrome*
    - X-linked recessive disorder with abnormal humoral and cell-mediated immunity
    - Seen usually in the 1st month of life in male children and is accompanied by bloody diarrhea, purpura

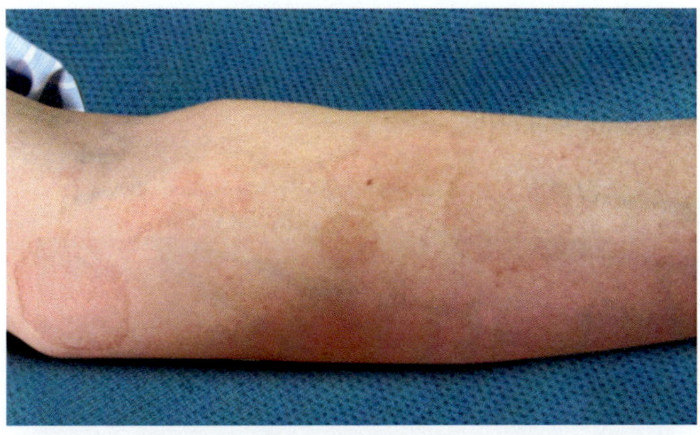

Fig. 4.14: Extensive patches of T, versicolor

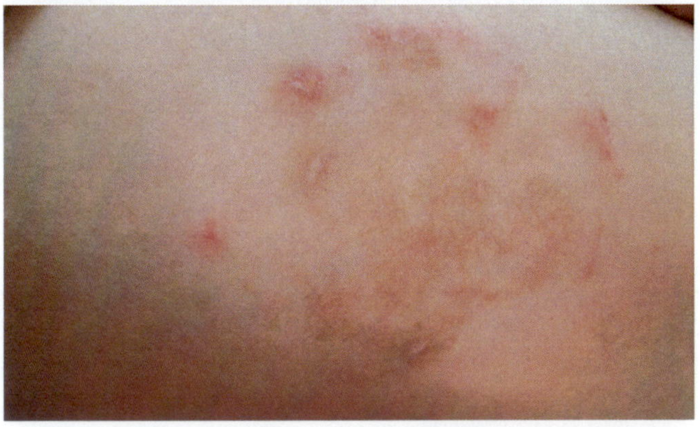

Fig. 4.15: Patch of T corporis modified by application of local steroid

and petechiae with a generalized rash identical to AD.[3]
- *Hyper IgE syndrome*
    ♦ Autosomal dominant disease with deficient Th1 response
    ♦ The child presents with a characteristic facies and abnormal dentition and a rash similar to AD mainly involving the scalp, axillae and groins
    ♦ Also accompanied by staphylococcal infections of the skin, lungs and sinuses
    ♦ Elevated levels of IgE and eosinophils are also found.
  - Di George syndrome
  - Severe combined immunodeficiency disease
- *Metabolic and nutritional diseases*
  - Phenylketonuria and Hartnup's disease
  - Niacin, zinc, pyridoxine deficiency.
- Graft versus host disease

- *Bullous diseases (Fig. 4.16)*
    – Bullous pemphigoid
    – Pemphigus foliaceus
- Drug eruptions (Fig. 4.17)
- Photodermatitis (Fig. 4.18).

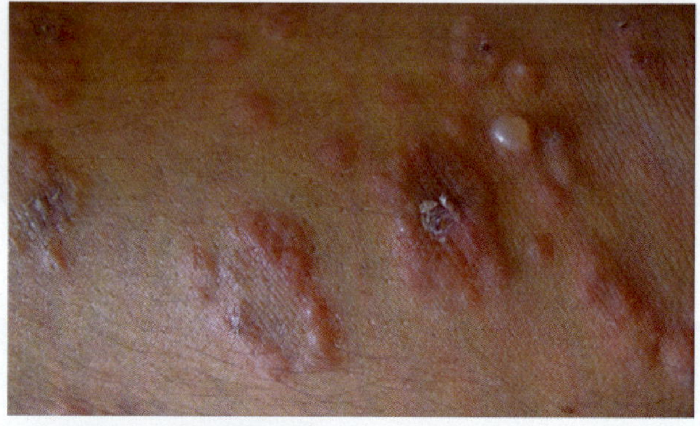

Fig. 4.16: Bullous disorders

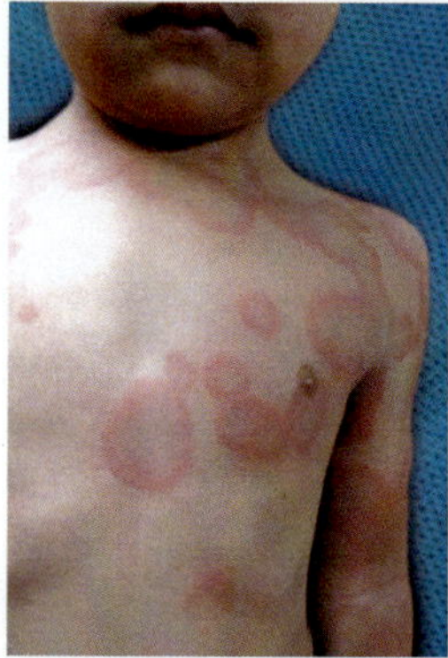

Fig. 4.17: Drug eruptions

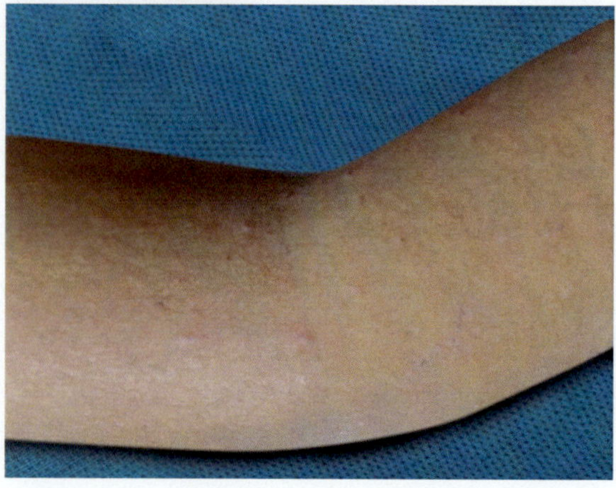

Fig. 4.18: Photodermatitis

REFERENCES

1. Dhar S, Banerjee R. Atopic dermatitis in infants and children in India. Indian J Dermatol Venereol Leprol. 2010;76:504-13.
2. Corominas M, et al. Predictors of atopy in HIV infected individuals. Ann Allergy Asthma Immunol. 2000;84:607.
3. Hochreutener H, Wuthrich B, Huwyler T, Schopler K, Seger R, Baerlocher K. Variant of hyper IgE syndrome: the differentiation from atopic dermatitis is important because of treatment and prognosis. Dermatologica. 1991;182:7-11.

SEVERITY OF DISEASE

MEASUREMENT OF DISEASE SEVERITY

Once the diagnosis of AD is made, various therapeutic options can be specifically selected depending on the disease severity. Even for experimental and investigational purposes, a specific severity measure can decide on the outcome of therapy.

Measuring the disease severity and its impact on the patient constitutes an important aspect in the management of AD for monitoring the response in everyday clinical practice and in clinical trials.

In this regard, various eczema severity scales were developed over years. The two most tested 'objective' clinical indices are the SCORAD index[1] and the Eczema Area and Severity index[2] (EASI).

Severity Scoring of Atopic Dermatitis Index (SCORAD)

The SCORAD index was introduced as a simple tool for the measurement of disease severity in clinical trials by the European Task Force on Atopic Dermatitis in 1983.[1] Here body diagrams are used to record the parameters. The following scores are taken and are added to each other.

- Six clinical signs (erythema, edema/papulation, oozing/crust, excoriation, lichenification, dryness of uninvolved area) are measured on a scale of 0–3 each measured at a representative body site
- The disease extent measured using the 'rule of nine'
- The above 2 are added to a visual analogue score for itch (0–10) and sleep loss (0–10) (maximum score-103)

The total scores are noted and the disease severity is assessed (Table 4.5).

Mild eczema was defined as SCORAD <15 and being transient. Moderate eczema was defined as SCORAD 15–40 and being recurrent; severe eczema as SCORAD >40 and being persistent.[1]

As this combines both objective (physician) and subjective (patient) parameters, it gives a complete assessment of the patient if correctly done.

Table 4.5: The SCORAD index	
Severity	*Scores*
Mild	<15
Moderate	15–40
Severe	>40

But this is not without disadvantages.
- There may be marked intra- and inter-observer variability in the interpretation
- Erythema assessment may be difficult in darker skin color.

A patient oriented PO-SCORAD which is a self-assessed version of SCORAD has also been described.[3]

EASI

- Was developed in 1998 as a tool for assessing the severity of AD and response to therapeutic interventions[4,5] (Table 4.6)
- Four clinical signs are assessed—erythema, induration/papulation, excoriation and lichenification on a scale of 0–3, each at four body sites
- Extent of the disease too assessed at these four sites
- There is a constant weighted value for multiplying in each region which represents the contribution of each mentioned body area to the total body surface area
- The sum of the scores for each body region are added and that gives the EASI total (maximum score-72)
- A multicenter study has shown the ease of administration and validity of the EASI score.[6]

Subsequently various other scoring systems were developed. Most of them appear to be modifications of early systems.
- The six area six sign atopic dermatitis (SASSAD) severity score[7] is a refinement of SCORAD which can be assessed quickly and easily.
- Modified Rajka and Langeland Severity Assessment (The Nottingham Eczema Severity score[8])
- The Assessment Measure for Atopic Dermatitis (ADAM)[9]
- Atopic Dermatitis Severity Index (ADASI)[10]
  - Was based on PASI, an index for psoriasis
- Patient Oriented Eczema Measure (POEM)
- The Three Item Severity Score (TIS)[11]
  - A simple scoring system compared to SCORAD and EASI which are time consuming
  - Based on the evaluation of erythema, edema/papulation and excoriation on a scale of 0–3.
  - Does not take into account the body surface area.

Schmitt et al.[12] assessed the validity, reliability, sensitivity to change and practical use of outcome measures for disease activity in AD. They assessed 20 outcome measures out of which SCORAD, EASI and POEM have been adequately validated and can be recommended for everyday clinical practice and even for clinical trials.

As far as Indian studies are concerned, the SCORAD index was used to measure the severity of the disease in a study. Two groups were taken, one consisting of children of Indian parents living in the UK and the US, the other with children born to parents living in India. 33 children in each group with similar age, sex and history of atopy for 3 years were taken. The mean severity scores were 8.64 among the cases and 6.34 in the controls, which was a statistically significant difference.[13]

REFERENCES

1. European Task Force on Atopic dermatitis. Severity scoring on atopic dermatitis: The SCORAD index. Dermatology. 1993;186: 23-31.
2. Darsow U, Wollenberg A, Simon D, et al. ETFAD/EADV eczema task force 2009 position paper on diagnosis and treatment of atopic dermatitis. J Eur Acad Dermatol Venereol. 2010;24:317-28.
3. Vourc`h-Jourdain M, Barbarot S, Taieb A, et al. Patient-Oriented SCORAD: A self-assessment score in atopic dermatitis. Dermatology. 2009;218:246-51.
4. Tofte S, Graeber M, Cherill R, et al. Eczema Area and Severity Index: a new tool to evaluate atopic dermatitis. J Eur Acad Dermatol Venereol. 1998;11(suppl 2):48.
5. Hanifin JM, Thurston M, Omoto M, et al. The EASI evaluator group. The Eczema Area and Severity Index (EASI): assessment of reliability in atopic dermatitis. Exp Dermatol. 2001;10:11-8.
6. Barbier N, Paul C, Luger T, et al. Validation of the eczema area and severity index for atopic dermatitis in a cohort of 1550 patients from the pimecrolimus cream 1% randomised control clinical trials programme. Br J Dermatol. 2004;150:96-102.
7. Berth-Jones J. Six Area Six Sign atopic dermatitis (SASSAD) severity score: A simple system for monitoring disease activity in atopic dermatitis. Br J Dermatol. 1996;135(Suppl 48):25-30.
8. Emmerson RM, Charman CR, Williams HC, et al. Modified Rajka and Langeland severity assessment (MRSA) for atopic dermatitis: a useful tool for epidemiological studies (abstract). Br J Dermatol. 1998;139(Suppl 51):65.
9. Charman D, Varigos G, Horne DJ, et al. The development of a practical and reliable assessment measure for atopic dermatitis (ADAM). J Outcome Meas. 1999;3:21-33.
10. Bahmer FA, Schafer J, Schubert HJ. Quantification of the extent and the severity of atopic dermatitis: The ADASI score. Arch dermatol. 1991;127:1239.
11. Wolkerstorfer A, Ward vanderSpek FB, Glazenburg EJ, et al. Scoring the severity of atopic dermatitis: Three Item Severity Score as a rough system for daily practice and as a pre-screening tool for studies. Acta Dermatol Venereol. 1999;79:356-9.
12. Schimitt J, Langan S, Williams HC. What are the best outcome measurements for atopic eczema? A systematic review. European Dermatolo-Epidemiology network. Allergy Clin Immunol. 2007;120:1389-98.
13. Dhar S, Banerjee R, Dutta AK, Gupta AB. Comparison between the severity of atopic dermatitis in Indian Children born and brought up in UK and USA and that of Indian children born and brought up in India. Indian J Dermatol. 2003;48:200-2.

QUALITY OF LIFE (QOL)

Skin sensitivity and skin-related quality of life (QOL) are massively impaired by chronic skin diseases.[1-3] Atopic dermatitis is one such condition where QOL gets greatly affected because of the severe itching, visible extensive skin lesions and above all, its involvement from a very early age. The child's scholastic performance can get adversely affected. Because of all these, the overall confidence of the child may be impaired.

Family gets adversely affected with a child being affected at home. Parents' sleep gets disturbed, holiday choices are restricted, food restrictions for the child alters the routine diet of the family and even relationships and social life may suffer.

Atopic dermatitis is a disease with a Th2-mediated immunological response predominating over Th1 response. Glucocorticoids released as a response to stress cultivate Th2 response while inhibiting Th1 response thus, aggravating atopic manifestations according to the recent research.[4] This indicates that it is a difficult disease to tackle with, a double edged sword where the disease causes stress and stress in turn causes aggravation of the disease.

It may reduce the patient's confidence to a great extent in the school or at work and even affect the interpersonal relationships.

Such patients tend to have a habitual scratching behavior, which should be called "addictive scratching" or "scratch dependence". This behavior worsens their eruption.[5]

A psychotherapist comes into play in this regard as counseling and therapy play an important role in helping the patients cope with the condition better.

The effects of psychological interventions have been studied in a few studies. A meta-analysis was published in 2007 by Chidaetal of 13 randomized control studies of the effectiveness of psychological interventions in patients with AD.[6]

QOL has been defined as 'the individual's perception of their position in life, in the context of culture and various systems in which they live, in relation to their goals, expectations, standards and concerns'.[7]

QOL assessment may contain both objective measures, which function on what an individual can do and are important in health measurement, and subjective measures, which reflect the meaning to the individual.[8]

Dermatological life quality index (DLQI) is one of the commonly used instruments for the measurement of QOL in AD patients. It is a tool specific to dermatological disorders which involves 10 items focused on six dimensions—symptoms, daily activities, leisure, work, personal relationships and treatment.[9] It is useful both in clinical practice and clinical trials.

There are various types of questionnaires available for measuring QOL in AD. Most of them contain questions regarding physical symptoms, social impact and emotion. Separate questionnaires are available for children and adults. QOL measurements are increasingly being added to many research studies on AD.

There are various other types of questionnaires available for measuring QOL in AD. Most of them contain questions regarding physical symptoms, social impact and emotion. Separate questionnaires are available for children and adults. QOL measurements are increasingly being added to many research studies on AD.

Parent's index of quality of life in atopic dermatitis (Pi QOL-AE) has been developed to measure the impact of AD in the child on parents.[10]

The children's dermatology life quality of index (CDLQI) is a tool developed for children to assess the impact of the disease in them.[11] This is for the age group 4–15. It is now available as a cartoon version which has been validated to the text-only-version.[12] This version was more acceptable by the children and was completed earlier than the text version.

The dermatitis family impact (DFI) questionnaire is a useful questionnaire to determine the ways in which the lives of parents of children with AD are affected[13] (maximum score -30).

REFERENCES

1. Harth W, Gieler U. Psychosomatische Dermatologie. Heidelberg: Springer; 2006. pp. 84-90.
2. Misery L, Finlay AY, Martin N, Boussettab S, Nguyenc C, Myonb E, et al. Atopic dermatitis: impact on the quality of life of patients and their partners. Dermatology. 2007;215:123-9.
3. Schmid-Ott G, Burchard R, Niederauer HH, Lamprecht F, Künsebeck HW. Stigmatisierungsgeñihl und Lebensqualitätbei Patient enmit Psoriasis und Atopic dermatitis. Hautarzt. 2003; 54:852-7.
4. Suárez AL, Feramisco JD, Koo J, Steinhoff M. Psycho-neuroimmunology of Psychological Stress and Atopic Dermatitis: Pathophysiologic and Therapeutic Updates. Acta Derm Venereol. 2012;92:7-15.
5. Kobayashi M. Investigation of scratching behavior in atopic dermatitis patients. Jpn J Dermatol. 2000;110:275-82. (In Japanese with English abstract.)
6. Chida Y, Steptoe A, Hirakawa N, Sudo N, Kubo C. The effects of psychological intervention on atopic dermatitis. Int Arch Allergy Immunol. 2007;144:1-9.
7. Schipper H, Clinch JJ, Olweny CLM. Quality of life studies: Definitions and conceptual frameworks. In: Spilker B (ed).

Quality of life and pharmacoeconomics in Clinical Trials, 2nd edn. Philadelphia: Lippincot-Raven; 1996.

8. Eiser C, Morse R. Can parents rate their child's health-related quality of life? Results of a systematic review. Qual life Res. 2001;10:347-57.

9. Finlay AY, Khan GK. Dermatology Life Quality Index (DLQI)–a simple practical measure for routine clinical use. Clin Exp Dermatol. 1994;19:210-6.

10. Whalley D, Huels L, McKenna SP, Van Assche D. The benefit of pimecrolimus (EledilSDZASM 981) on parents' quality of life in the treatment of pediatric atopic dermatitis. Pediatrics. 2002;110:1133-6.

11. Lewis –Jones MS, Finlay AY. The Childrens' Dermatology Life Quality Index: The initial validation and practical use. Br J Dermatol. 1995;132;942-9.

12. Holme SA, Man I, Sharpe JL, Dykes PJ, Lewis –Jones MS, Finlay AY. The Childrens' Dermatology Life Quality Index; validation of the cartoon version. Br J Dermatol. 1993;148;285-90.

13. Lawson V, Lewis-Jones MS, Finlay AY, Reid P, Owens RG. The family impact of childhood atopic dermatitis: the Dermatitis Family Impact questionnaire. Br J Dermatol. 1998;138:107-13.

Management of Atopic Dermatitis

Shaurya Rohatgi, Satish Udare

AIM OF TREATMENTS

Barrier repair: Moisturizers, bathing practices, wet-wrap therapy.

Topical anti-inflammatory therapy: Topical corticosteroids, topical calcineurin inhibitors, tar preparation, topical antimicrobials and antiseptics.

Systemic Therapy: Cyclosporine, azathioprine, methotrexate, mycophenolate mofetil, systemic corticosteroids, omalizumab, other biological agents, interferon gamma, intravenous immunoglobulin, antimicrobials.

Antipruritic therapy: Topical antipruritic agents, ultraviolet (UV) therapy, oral antihistamines, other systemic anti-pruritic agents.

Nonpharmacologic interventions: Dietary interventions and supplements, psychodermatological aspects and psychological interventions, environmental modifications, educational interventions, complementary and alternative medicine.

MANAGEMENT

Atopic dermatitis (AD) is a chronic, pruritic inflammatory skin disease that occurs most frequently in children, but also affects many adults. The relapsing nature of this disorder results in significant morbidity and adversely affects quality of life of patients and their families.[1] It is a multifaceted condition presenting therapeutic challenge as it is not curable. Accordingly, the primary objective of treatment is achieving the following two scenarios:

- To make the patient asymptomatic or mildly symptomatic, so that the disease causes no interference in the patient's day to day life. In addition, keep the dependence on drugs minimal and avoid and treat complications
- Once the disease is controlled, limit the acute or intense exacerbations to a minimum. Even if an exacerbation occurs, see to it that it is not severe or protracted.

Education and Counseling

Educating the patients and family members is an important aspect, but often neglected while treating AD. Information about the chronic nature of the disease, exacerbating factors, the need for continued adherence to proper skin care practices and need for compliance to appropriate treatment options, including discussion of side effects and potency of topical corticosteroids is imperative in order to achieve effective control of disease. The evidence roots from the effectiveness of educational strategies in improving disease severity and treatment adherence in studies of nurse-led educational sessions and multidisciplinary parent-education programs.[2,3]

Written information that includes detailed skin-care recommendations and methods for environmental control can be helpful. Written plans should include guidelines on how to monitor AD, how to respond to changes in disease status, and when to seek additional medical help.[4]

BARRIER REPAIR

Topical agents are the mainstay of AD therapy. Agents from several classes are frequently used in combination, because they address different aspects of AD pathogenesis. Even in more severe cases needing systemic or phototherapy, they are often used in conjunction with these modalities.[5]

Moisturizers and Treatment of Epidermal Barrier Defect

Moisturizers

Moisturizers can be broadly classified into 3 types (Table 5.1). Varothai et al.[6] has reviewed the efficacy of moisturizers in AD.

A dysfunctional epidermal barrier is seen in AD resulting in xerosis as the clinical manifestation. The application of moisturizers increases hydration of the skin,[7,8] aid in restoring the impaired barrier function of the epidermis, lessen symptoms and signs of AD, including pruritus, erythema, fissuring, and lichenification,[7,8,9] increases the efficacy of topical corticosteroids, and also have a steroid-sparing action.[9,10]

Moisturizers can be the main primary treatment for mild disease and should be part of the regimen for moderate and severe disease.[11] They are also an important component of maintenance treatment and prevention of flares. Moisturizers are therefore a cornerstone of AD therapy and should be included in all management plans.[5]

Anti-inflammatory agents are added into some more sophisticated moisturizers to alleviate atopic xerosis and

Table 5.1: Classification of moisturizers

Type	Mechanism of action	Examples
Emollient	Lubricate and soften the skin	Lauric acid, linoleic acid, linolenic acid, oleic acid, stearic acid
Occlusive	Form a hydrophobic film to retard evaporation of water	Beeswax, carnauba, lanolin, mineral oils, paraffin, petrolatum, propylene glycol, silicones, squalene
Humectant	Attract and hold water	Alpha hydroxy acids, glycerin, hyaluronic acid, propylene glycol, pyrrolidone, carboxylic acid, sorbitol, sugars

mild AD without topical corticosteroids treatment.[6] Aloe vera, chamomile oil (*Matricaria chamomilla*), St. John's wort (*Hypericum perforatum*), grape-seed extract (*Vitis vinifera*), shea butter, licochalcone, ceramide, nicotinamide, and palmitoylethanolamine are some of the agents which are increasingly being used as additives to increase the efficacy of moisturizers.[6] Sole use of emollients without sufficient topical anti-inflammatory therapy involves a considerable risk for disseminated bacterial and viral infection, which is already increased in AD patients.[12] The disadvantage is affordability in the Indian setting which limits the clinician from prescribing such sophisticated moisturizers.

Moisturizers should have the following basic ingredients in optimum concentrations:

- **Water:** 65–85% (lotions and creams)—Water forms the base which dilutes as well as disperses the various ingredients following which it evaporates from the skin surface
- **Lipids:** 5–35% (lotions and creams), up to 100% (ointments)—Lipids (mineral oil, petrolatum, lanolin, beeswax, vegetable oils, fatty alcohols, ceramides) have an occlusive effect to prevent water loss, helps to repair lipid layers in the epidermis, thus restoring barrier function of skin.
- **Emulsifiers (1–2%):** Emulsifiers (stearic acid, triethanolamine, quaternium-15) are required to allow water and lipids to stay in suspension.
- **Active ingredients (0.05–15%):** Modern day moisturizers have a variety of additives (glycerine, dimethicone, allantoin, urea, AHAs, lactic acid, filaggrin degradation products, sunscreens) each serving a unique function (e.g. attract water to the skin, skin protectants, fill in spaces between cells, replace amino acids, physiological lipids, block UV)
- Preservatives (0.1–1%): Preservatives (parabens, disodium EDTA, methylisothiazolinones prevent the growth of microorganisms within the product
- Fragrance (<0.25%): May be added to mask the odor of lipids or impart scent.

It is also imperative to add that in our opinion, an ideal moisturizer should be free of fragrance, color or preservative but in current market perspective, this is impractical. It should offer protection against environmental factors with no negative effects on barrier maturation. The sensitization potential and systemic effect should be negligible and last but not the least, cosmetic acceptance should be optimal.

In the lack of systematic studies to define an optimal amount or frequency of application of moisturizers,[13] experience dictates that liberal and frequent reapplication is necessary such that xerosis is minimal.[5] European guidelines[14] recommend a minimum of 250 g per week of emollient cream/ointment.

Bathing Practices

Bathing can have a beneficial as well as a detrimental effect on the patient's skin depending on the manner in which it is carried out.

Hydration of the skin and removal of scale, crust, irritants, and allergens is facilitated by bathing which can be helpful in AD.[15] However, if the water is left to evaporate from the skin, greater transepidermal water loss occurs.[16] Therefore, application of moisturizers soon after bathing is necessary to maintain good hydration status.[16,17] It is recommended that up to once-daily bathing be performed to remove serous crust, as long as moisturizers follow as above; the duration should be limited to short periods of time (e.g. 5–10 minutes) with use of warm water.[5]

If there are areas of significantly inflamed skin, soaking in plain water for 20 minutes followed by the immediate application of pharmacologic anti-inflammatory therapies (e.g. topical corticosteroids [TCS]) to these sites, without toweling dry, is a helpful treatment measure. This "soak and smear" technique can improve response in cases where the topical anti-inflammatory alone is inadequate.[15]

Limited use of nonsoap cleansers that are neutral to low pH, hypoallergenic and fragrance free is recommended. Soaps consist of surfactants that interact with stratum corneum proteins and lipids, but in a manner that causes damage, dry skin and irritation.[18,19] Most soap are alkaline in pH, whereas the skin's normal pH is 4–5.5 (Figure 5.1). Instead, nonsoap-based surfactants and synthetic detergents (syndets) are often recommended for better tolerance.[20,21]

Data are limited on the addition of oils, emollients and other related additives to bath water and their benefits for AD.[22] No published RCTs have tested the clinical benefit of combining bath emollients with directly-applied emollients after bathing. However, twice weekly bleach baths, i.e. adding sodium

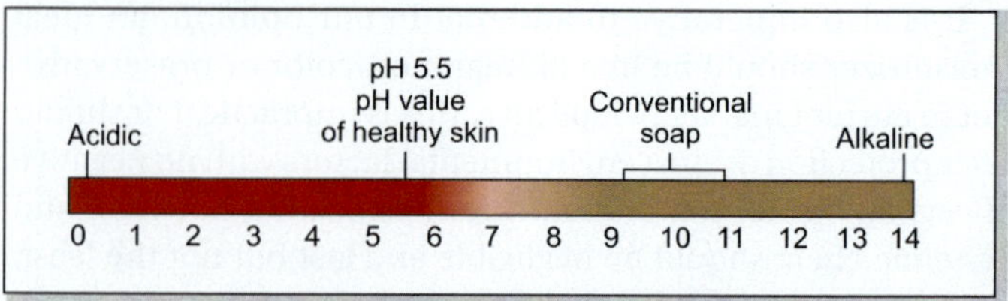

Fig. 5.1: Soap and skin pH

hypochlorite to the bath-water inhibits bacterial count and may be advised to every treatment in AD especially in patients with recurrent skin infections.[4,14]

Wet-wrap Therapy

Wet-wrap therapy (WWT) is one method to quickly reduce AD severity, and is often used in the setting of significant flares and/or recalcitrant disease. In this technique, a topical agent is covered by a wetted first layer of tubular bandages, gauze, or a cotton suit, followed by a dry second/outside layer. WWT appears to help via occluding the topical agent for increased penetration, decreasing water loss, and providing a physical barrier against scratching. The wrap can be worn from several hours to 24 hours at a time, depending on patient tolerance. Most suggest several days of use, although a few studies continued WWT for up to 2 weeks.[23,24]

Topical anti-inflammatory Therapy

European guidelines[14] advocate the application of topical anti-inflammatory agents on hydrated skin, especially when using ointments. The emollient should be applied first when it is a cream, 15 min before the anti-inflammatory topical is applied and when it is an ointment 15 min after. In view of the authors, the practicality of this method in terms of time consumed for treatment is a concern.

Application amount of topical anti-inflammatory therapy should follow the finger-tip unit (FTU) rule (Table 5.2).[14] A FTU (Figure 5.2) is the amount of ointment expressed from a tube with a 5-mm diameter nozzle and measured from the distal skin-crease to the tip of the index finger (~0.5 g); this is an adequate amount for application to two adult palm areas, which is approximately 2% of an adult body surface area.

Topical Corticosteroids

TCS are the mainstay of anti-inflammatory therapy in AD. TCS are grouped into 7 classes, from very low/lowest potency

Table 5.2: Fingertip unit

Area that needs treatment	FTUs (adults)	FTUs (children 1–2 years)
Face and neck	2.5	1.5
One hand and fingers	1	0.5
One arm, hand and fingers	4	1.5
Chest and abdomen	7	2
Back and buttocks	7	3
One leg and foot	8	2
FTU: Finger tip unit		

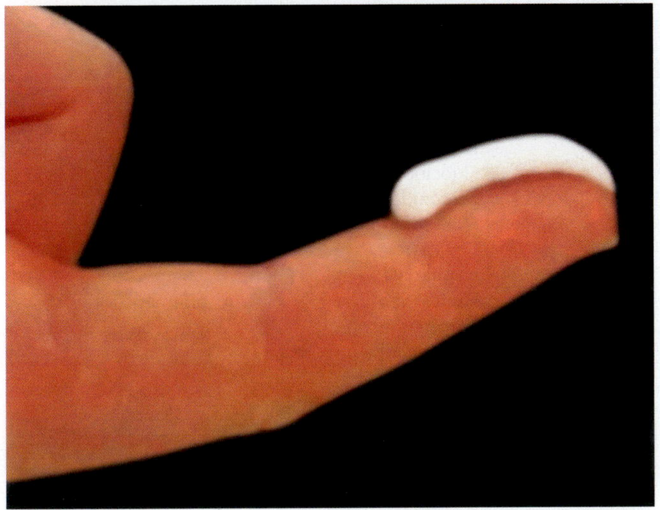

Fig. 5.2: One fingertip unit

(VII) to very high potency (I), based on vasoconstriction assays (Table 5.3).

Corticosteroids (CS) mediate their anti-inflammatory effects through a cytoplasmic glucocorticoid receptor (GCR) in target cells. Upon ligand binding, the CS/GCR complex translocates into the nucleus where it mediates its anti-inflammatory effects via two major actions.[25]

1. *Transactivation* is the process which induces gene transcription through binding of GCR dimers to glucocorticoid response elements in the promoter regions of target genes. This is mainly responsible for the unwanted side effects of CS.
2. *Transrepression* the mechanism responsible for the anti-inflammatory effects, which is independent of GCR DNA binding. In this process, ligand-bound GCR binds to various transcription factors, including activator protein-1

Table 5.3: Relative potencies of topical corticosteroids			
I. Very high potency	Clobetasol propionate	Cream, foam, ointment	0.05
	Diflorasone diacetate	Ointment	0.05
	Halobetasol propionate	Cream, ointment	0.05
II. High potency	Augmented betamethasone dipropionate	Cream	0.05
	Betamethasone dipropionate	Cream, foam, ointment, solution	0.05
	Desoximetasone	Cream, ointment	0.25
	Desoximetasone	Gel	0.05
	Fluocinonide	Cream, gel, ointment	0.05
	Halcinonide	Solution cream	0.1
	Mometasone furoate	Ointment	0.1
	Triamcinolone acetonide	Ointment	0.5
		Cream, ointment	
III-IV. Medium potency	Betamethasone valerate	Cream, foam, lotion, ointment	0.1
	Desoximetasone	Cream	0.05
	Fluocinolone acetonide	Cream, ointment	0.025
	Flurandrenolide	Cream, ointment	0.05
	Fluticasone propionate	Cream	0.05
	Fluticasone propionate	Ointment	0.005
	Mometasone furoate	Cream	0.1
	Triamcinolone acetonide	Cream, ointment	0.1
V. Lower-medium potency	Hydrocortisone butyrate	Cream, ointment, solution cream	0.1
	Hydrocortisone probutate	Cream, ointment	0.1
	Hydrocortisone valerate		0.2
VI. Low potency	Desonide	Cream, gel, foam	0.05
	Fluocinolone acetonide	Ointment cream, solution	0.01
VII. Lowest potency	Dexamethasone	Cream	0.1
	Hydrocortisone	Cream, lotion	0.25, 0.5, 1
	Hydrocortisone acetate	Ointment, solution cream, ointment	0.5–1

and NF-κB, via protein-protein interactions to inhibit the transcriptional activity of various proinflammatory genes encoding proinflammatory proteins, such as cytokines (IL-1, IL-2, IL-3, IL-4, IL-5, IL-6, IL-11, IL-13, TNF-α, and GM-CSF), chemokines (IL-8, RANTES, macrophage inflammatory protein–1α [MIP-1a], monocyte chemotactic protein-1 [MCP-1], MCP-3, MCP-4, and eotaxin), and adhesion molecules (ICAM-1, VCAM-1, and E-selectin).

No comprehensive evidence was identified comparing TCS with each other in terms of effectiveness.[5,26] A stepped/matched approach consists of matching potency of TCS with severity of the eczema: mild-potency TCS for mild disease, moderate potency for moderate disease and potent or ultra-high potent TCS reserved for short term use in severe eczema.[27] The choice of TCS potency should also be tailored to the age of the patient, the body region being treated, and the degree to which the skin is inflamed. For delicate areas of skin, such as the face and flexures, only mild or moderately potent preparations should be used.[26]

A proportionately greater body surface area to weight ratio in children result in a higher degree of absorption for the same applied amount of TCS. But during significant acute flares, the use of mid- or higher-potency TCS for short courses may be appropriate to gain rapid control of symptoms, even in children.[28,29] However, for long-term management, the least-potent corticosteroid that is effective should be used to minimize the risk of adverse effects.[5]

Generally, the recommended frequency of TCS application is twice daily, but evidence suggests that once-daily application of some potent corticosteroids may be as effective as twice-daily application.[30] Patients should be advised to continue with emollient therapy during treatment with topical corticosteroids.[26]

Vehicle is also an important consideration with regard to choice of TCS. Ointments are used in lichenified areas where increased penetration and higher potency is required. Creams are used for non-lichenified areas whereas lotions and gels are best suited for intertriginous and hairy areas.

Cutaneous side effects include purpura, telangiectasia, striae, focal hypertrichosis, and acneiform or rosacea-like eruptions. Of greatest concern is skin atrophy, which can be induced by any TCS, though higher-potency agents, occlusion, use on thinner skin, and older patient age increase this risk.[31] Continuous application of TCS for long periods of time should be avoided, to limit the occurrence of negative changes. Proactive, once to twice weekly application of mid-potency TCS for up to 40 weeks has not demonstrated these adverse events in clinical trials.[32] Topically-applied corticosteroids, particularly high- and very high–potency agents, can be absorbed at a degree sufficient to cause systemic side effects. The risk of hypothalamic-pituitary-adrenal axis suppression is low but increases with prolonged continuous use, especially in individuals receiving corticosteroids concurrently in other forms (inhaled, intranasal, or oral).[33] As discussed above, children are more susceptible as a result of a greater body surface to weight ratio. Nonetheless, a systematic review did conclude that TCS overall have a good safety profile.[31] Moreover, the American Academy of Dermatology recommends no specific monitoring for systemic side effects for patients with AD at this time.[5]

Although judicious use of TCS is certainly warranted, recognition of undertreatment as a result of steroid phobia is also important.[5] Surveys have shown patient's concern about use of TCS on their own or their child's skin, noncompliance with therapy as a result of these concerns[34] and poor knowledge of steroid class potencies leading to inappropriate use.[35] In the Indian setting, where steroid abuse is rampant, adverse effects from improper use is more of a concern rather than steroid phobia. Therefore, counseling and educating the patient about the use of steroids is of utmost importance.

Topical Calcineurin Inhibitors

Two TCI are available, topical tacrolimus ointment (0.03% and 0.1% strengths) and pimecrolimus cream (1% strength). The anti-inflammatory potency of 0.1% tacrolimus ointment is similar to a corticosteroid with moderate potency,[36] whereas 1% pimecrolimus cream is less active.[37] Tacrolimus is approved for moderate to severe disease, whereas pimecrolimus is indicated for mild to moderate AD, and 6-week comparative studies support a greater effect for tacrolimus over this time period for all AD severities.[38,39]

FDA approves TCI as second-line therapy for the short-term and noncontinuous chronic treatment of AD in nonimmunocompromised individuals who have failed to respond adequately to other topical prescription treatments for AD, or when those treatments are not advisable.[5] TCI have the benefit of not carrying risk for cutaneous atrophy, with little negative effect on collagen synthesis and skin thickness. TCI can therefore be used as steroid-sparing agents and long-term studies have shown that they do reduce the need for TCS use.[40] They have also been demonstrated to be more effective in reversing skin atrophy than vehicle.[41] TCI have particular use at sensitive skin sites, such as the face and skin folds, where there is a greater adverse risk profile with TCS.[5]

FDA approves use of tacrolimus 0.03% ointment and pimecrolimus cream for individuals' age 2 years and older, whereas tacrolimus 0.1% strength is only approved in those older than 15 years.[5] However, evidence from clinical trials supports the safe and effective use of topical tacrolimus 0.03% and pimecrolimus in children younger than 2 years, including in infants.[42]

Twice-daily applications of TCI are significantly more effective than vehicle or once-daily application[43,44] Moreover, intermittent application of TCI 2–3 times weekly to recurrent sites of disease has also been shown to be effective in reducing relapses.[45,46]

Common side effects include stinging and burning, which tend to lessen after several applications or when first preceded by a short period of topical steroid use. Allergic contact dermatitis and a rosacea-like granulomatous reaction have been reported.[5] The effect of continuation of TCI treatment on infected lesions has not been studied, but the prescribing information advocates against their use during acute infection.[5] Although, rare cases of malignancy have been reported a causal relationship has not been established. Moreover, interim analyses of ongoing, 10-year surveillance studies have not found any evidence to support these risks.[47]

Tar Preparation

Although tar preparations are widely used in the treatment of AD, there are no randomized controlled studies that have demonstrated their efficacy.[48,49] Newer coal tar products have been developed that are more cosmetically acceptable, with respect to odor and staining of clothes, than some older products.[50]

Bedtime application is recommended to enhance compliance. Odor during the day and staining of daytime clothing is limited due to removal of the drug during bath .[4] It is advisable not to use tar preparations on acutely inflamed skin because this can result in additional skin irritation. The theoretic risk of tar being a carcinogen may have been refuted by a sufficiently powered cohort analysis of both patients with psoriasis and those with eczema treated with tar which found no increased risk of malignancies.[51] Adverse effects associated with tars include folliculitis and, occasionally, photosensitivity. Tar shampoos are often beneficial when AD involves the scalp.[4]

Topical Antimicrobials and Antiseptics

A compromised physical barrier, diminished immune recognition and impaired antimicrobial peptide production predisposes atopic individuals to skin infections, particularly *Staphylococcus aureus* colonization. However, except for bleach baths with intranasal mupirocin, no topical antistaphylococcal treatment has been shown to be clinically helpful in patients with AD, and is not routinely recommended.[5]

PHOTOTHERAPY

Numerous studies have established the role of phototherapy in the treatment of AD and it represents a standard second-line treatment.[52] It can be used as monotherapy or in combination with emollients and topical steroids.[53] However, its use with TCI is cautioned, as the manufacturers suggest limiting exposure to natural and artificial light sources while using these topical medications.[54,55] The use of light therapy may decrease the need for topical steroid and topical immunomodulator use.[53]

Phototherapy can be administered in the form of natural sunlight, narrowband (NB) UVB, BB-UVB, UVA, topical and systemic psoralen plus UVA (PUVA), UVA and UVB (UVAB).[53] In the paucity of head-to-head trials, it is difficult to comment on the superiority of one over the other, although natural sunlight is likely less effective than artificial light sources.[52] UVA phototherapy and UVAB phototherapy have increased risks of side effects and UVAB is of limited availability. NB-UVB (Table 5.4) is generally the most commonly recommended light treatment on basis of its low-risk profile, relative efficacy, availability, and provider comfort level.[53] In addition, extracorporeal photochemotherapy has been used in patients with generalized and erythrodermic AD but response has been variable.[56] In the paucity of data, use of lasers are not recommended.[53]

Several common adverse effects[53] **include:** Actinic damage, local erythema and tenderness, pruritus, burning, and stinging. Less common consequences of light therapy include: Nonmelanoma skin cancer, melanoma (particularly with the use of PUVA), lentigines, photosensitive eruptions (especially polymorphous light eruption), folliculitis, photo-onycholysis, herpes simplex virus (HSV) reactivation, and facial hypertrichosis. Cataract formation is a recognized side effect specific to UVA therapy, whereas the addition of oral psoralen to UVA treatment frequently causes patients to have headaches, nausea, and vomiting, and rarely hepatotoxicity. Oral psoralen also increases a patient's photosensitivity, both cutaneous and ocular, for several hours after ingestion.

SYSTEMIC THERAPY

Systemic therapy is indicated and recommended in AD for patients in whom optimized topical regimens and/or phototherapy do not adequately control the disease, or when QOL is substantially impacted.[53] Prevailing literature suggests that cyclosporine, methotrexate (MTX), mycophenolate mofetil (MMF), and azathioprine (AZA) are used the most and are more efficacious in treating AD, whereas other agents (leukotriene

Table 5.4: Dosing guidelines for narrowband ultraviolet B

a. According to skin type

Skin type	Initial UVB dose, mJ/cm²	UVB increase after each treatment, mJ/cm²	Maximum dose, mJ/cm²
I	130	15	2000
II	220	25	2000
III	260	40	3000
IV	330	45	3000
V	350	60	5000
VI	400	65	5000

b. According to MED

Initial UVB	50% of MED
Treatments 1–20	Increase by 10% of initial MED
Treatment ≥21	Increase as ordered by physician

c. If subsequent treatments are missed for

4–7 days	Keep dose same
1–2 weeks	Decrease dose by 25%
2–3 weeks	Decrease dose by 50% or start over
3–4 weeks	Start over

d. Maintenance therapy for NB-UVB after >95% clearance

1x/week	NB-UVB for 4 week	Keep dose same
1x/2 week	NB-UVB for 4 week	Decrease dose by 25%
1x/4 week	NB-UVB	50% of highest dose

Administered 3–5 times/week

Because there is broad range of minimal erythema dose (MED) for NB-UVB by skin type, MED testing is generally recommended. It is critically important to meter UVB machine once weekly. UVB lamps steadily lose power. If UV output is not periodically measured and actual output calibrated into machine, clinician may have false impression that patient can be treated with higher doses when machine is actually delivering much lower dose than number entered. Minimum frequency of phototherapy sessions required per week for successful maintenance and length of maintenance period varies tremendously between individuals. Above table represents most ideal situation where patient can taper off phototherapy. In reality, many patients require 13/week NB-UVB phototherapy indefinitely for successful long-term maintenance.

Abbreviations: MED, minimal erythema dose; NB, narrowband; UV, ultraviolet.
Reprinted with permission.[57]

inhibitors, oral calcineurin inhibitors) have limited data (Table 5.5).[53] Biologic drugs, such as omalizumab are relatively new and further studies will consolidate its role in AD management. Although used frequently and shown to temporarily suppress disease, the AAD recommends avoidance of systemic corticosteroids due to the associated short- and long-term adverse effects and an overall unfavorable risk-benefit profile.[53]

Cyclosporine

Cyclosporin A (CSA) is an effective off-label treatment option for patients with AD refractory to conventional topical treatment.[53] CSA induces a significant decrease in disease activity within 2–6 weeks of treatment initiation.[48,58] A dosage of 3–6 mg/kg/d in pediatric age group and 150–300 mg/d in adults is used for AD treatment. Reports suggest that higher initial doses result in more rapid control of the disease and involved body surface area while improving QOL measures, such as pruritus and sleep disturbance. Although relapse after discontinuation of therapy is often observed, post-treatment disease severity often does not return to baseline levels.[59,60] The dosing regimens should be tailored on an individual basis aiming for the shortest possible treatment period, followed by maintenance of remission via emollients, topical agents, and/ or phototherapy.[61]

Azathioprine

AZA is recommended as a systemic agent for the treatment of refractory AD.[53] The usual dose range of 1–3 mg/kg/d has been used in AD. A delayed effect may be noted, with some patients needing 12 weeks or greater of medication to achieve full clinical benefit. Once clearance or near-clearance is achieved and maintained, AZA should be tapered or discontinued, with maintenance of remission via emollients and topical agents.[53]

Methotrexate

Once again, MTX is recommended as a systemic agent for the treatment of refractory AD.[53] A dose of 10–22.5 mg/week over a 24-week period attained good results.[62]

Mycophenolate Mofetil

Although the data is variable and efficacy is inconsistent, it overall suggests that MMF is an alternative therapy for refractory AD.[53] Usual dose ranges between 0.5 and 3 g/d.

Systemic Corticosteroids

Systemic steroids rapidly improve clinical symptoms of AD, however rebound flare and increased disease severity is a commonly observed phenomenon upon discontinuation.[53,61] In spite of temporary effectiveness, it is advisable to avoid systemic steroids for treatment of AD because the potential short- and long-term adverse effects largely outweigh the benefits. Systemic steroids may be considered for short-term use in individual cases where other systemic or phototherapy regimens are being initiated and/or optimized.[53,61]

Omalizumab

Omalizumab, a humanized IgG1 monoclonal antibody against IgE, has been tested in patients of AD refractory to conventional therapy. In contrast to patients with severe asthma and chronic idiopathic urticaria that showed significant improvement in their disease, it has failed to provide consistent significant clinical effects in most patients with AD.[63] Further studies are required to consolidate its role in the management of AD.

Other Biological Agents[63]

Although the results are conflicting and further studies are required to consolidate the findings, preliminary or theoretical data points out to the possible utility of other biologicals in the treatment of AD.

Small studies of rituximab, an antibody against CD20 that depletes B cells, have shown both positive and negative findings.[64,65] Anti-TNF agents (etanercept, infliximab) proved disappointing possibly because TNF-induced inflammatory responses have only a minor role in AD. Mepolizumab, a fully humanized, monoclonal antibody against IL-5, did not show clinical efficacy in patients with AD. Tocilizumab, an IL-6 receptor antagonist, has shown good result in 3 patients. Therapeutics that target IL-4 receptor (pascolizumab), IL-31, IL-17 or its receptor (ixekizumab, brodalumab, or AIN457), IL23 (MK-3222) or Th17 and Th22 pathways (ustekinumab) have theoretical potential for use in AD patients but have not been tried in AD.

Interferon Gamma

IFN gamma (IFN-γ) is a TH1 cytokine which has been shown to antagonize TH2 immune responses in vitro. Thrice weekly subcutaneous injections of 50 mg/m^2 showed significant improvement of AD in some studies.[66,67] But the high rate of unwanted drug effects, such as headache, muscle pain and fever and the high treatment cost are limiting the potential use of IFN-γ in chronic diseases.[68] The European guidelines do not recommend the use of IFN-γ for treatment of AD.[68] However, American guidelines recommend its use based on limited-quality evidence.[53]

Table 5.5: Dosing and monitoring guidelines for the use of selected systemic agents

Drug	Dosing	Baseline Monitoring	Follow-up monitoring	Miscellaneous
Cyclosporine	150–300 mg/d Pediatric: 3–6 mg/kg/d	Blood pressure x 2 Measurements, Renal function, Urinalysis with microscopic analysis, Fasting lipid profile CBC/differential/platelets Liver function, Mg, K, Uric acid, TB testing, HIV, if indicated, HCG, if indicated	Blood pressure every visit Every 2 weeks for 2–3 months, then monthly: Renal function, liver function, lipids, CBC/ differential/ platelets, Mg, K, uric acid If dose increased, check laboratory results 2–4 week after HCG, if indicated Annual TB testing	If Cr increases >25% above baseline, reduce dose by 1 mg/kg/d for 2–4 weeks and recheck; stop CSA if Cr remains >25% above baseline; hold at lower dose if level is within 25% of baseline Whole-blood CSA trough level in children if inadequate clinical response or concomitant use of potentially interacting medications
Azathioprine	1–3 mg/kg/d Pediatric: 1–4 mg/kg/d	Baseline TPMT CBC/differential/platelets Renal function, Liver function Hepatitis B and C TB testing HIV, if indicated HCG, if indicated	CBC/differential/platelets, liver function, renal function twice/ months x 2 months, monthly x 4 months, then every other month and with dose increases HCG, if indicated Annual TB testing	Dosing may be guided by TPMT enzyme activity

Drug	Dosing	Baseline Monitoring	Follow-up monitoring	Miscellaneous
Methotrexate	7.5–25 mg/week Pediatric: 0.2–0.7 mg/kg/week Consider test dose: 1.25–5 mg	CBC/differential/platelets Liver function Renal function Hepatitis B and C TB testing HIV, if indicated HCG, if indicated Pulmonary function tests, if indicated	CBC/differential/platelets, liver function weekly for 2–4 week and 1 week after each major dose increase, then every 2 week for 1 month and every 2–3 months while on stable doses Renal function every 6–12 months Annual TB testing HCG as indicated	Liver enzymes transiently increase after MTX dosing; obtain laboratory results 5–7 d after the last dose Significant elevations of liver enzymes: - Exceeding x2 normal, check more frequently - Exceeding x3 normal, reduce the dose and recheck - Exceeding x5 normal, discontinue Avoid in patients at risk for hepatotoxicity Liver biopsy may be considered at 3.5–4.0 g of cumulative MTX in adults No standard liver biopsy recommendations for children Consider pulmonary function tests before initiation and during therapy in consultation with a pulmonologist for patients with asthma or chronic cough, or consider alternative therapies CXR if respiratory symptoms arise
Mycophenolate mofetil	1.0–1.5 g orally twice daily Pediatric: 1200 mg/m^2 daily, which corresponds to 30–50 mg/kg/d	CBC/differential/platelets Renal function Liver function TB testing HIV, if indicated HCG, if indicated	CBC/differential/platelets, liver function every 2 weeks for 1 month; then monthly for 3 months; then every 2–3 months thereafter HCG if indicated Annual TB testing	

Abbreviations: CBC, Complete blood cell count; Cr, creatinine; CSA, cyclosporine; CXR, chest radiograph; HCG, human chorionic gonadotropin; K1, potassium; Mg1, magnesium; MTX, methotrexate; TB, tuberculosis; TPMT, thiopurine methyltransferase. Reprinted with permission[53].

Intravenous Immunoglobulin

In addition to its immunomodulatory activity, intravenous immunoglobulin (Iv-Ig) contain high concentrations of staphylococcal toxin–specific antibodies which can interact directly with microbes or toxins involved in the pathogenesis of this disease.[69] However, treatment of severe refractory AD with Iv-Ig has yielded conflicting results.[70] In view of insufficient data, American guidelines do not recommend the use of Iv-Ig for the treatment of AD.[53]

Antimicrobials

Although *S. Aureus* can be cultured from greater than 90% of adult patients with AD,[71] most patients do not show increased morbidity from this colonization. The catch lies in the similar clinical appearance of active localized infection and active AD posing a diagnostic conundrum.[53] While both show oozing, weeping and crusting, presence of purulent exudate and pustules swings the pendulum in favor of secondary bacterial infection over inflammation from dermatitis. A less common complication due to HSV infection called "eczema herpeticum," can present a challenge due to increased patient morbidity.

Routine use of systemic antibiotics in the treatment of noninfected AD is not recommended, except in patients with clinical evidence of bacterial infection. Antibiotics may be administered in addition to standard, suitable treatment for AD, including the concurrent application of topical steroids.[71,72] Similarly, eczema herpeticum should be treated with systemic antiviral agents.

ANTIPRURITIC THERAPY

Antipruritic therapy in AD is multidimensional treating the symptom itself, the contributing factors, such as dry skin, inflammation and the related scratch lesions. Pruritus can have a deleterious effect on the QOL of patients suffering from AD,[73,74] but very few studies have solely addressed antipruritic affect of therapeutic agents.[14]

Topical Antipruritic Agents

Anti-inflammatory agents, such as TCS and TCI have a rapid antipruritic effect in AD. In addition to management of eczematous lesions, antipruritic effect of TCS can be used in the initial phase of AD exacerbation and that of TCI until clearance of eczema.[14] Moisturizers also help to alleviate itch by reducing dryness.

The antipruritic effect of local anesthetics was demonstrated in AD, but controlled clinical trials are pending. Therefore, routine clinical use in AD cannot be recommended as an adjuvant antipruritic therapy in AD.[14]

Eberlein et al. reported a 60% reduction in pruritus and the need to use corticosteroids in AD patients with the use of topical N-palmitoylethanolamine which is a cannabinoid receptor agonist.[75] Capsaicin exerts its functions via binding to transient receptor potential channel vanilloid (TRPV1) receptors which is located on free nerve endings. Repeated application of topical capsaicin releases and prevents specifically the reaccumulation of neuropeptides in unmyelinated, polymodal C-type cutaneous nerves. It has been shown to be effective for control of pruritus in AD.[76] Drake et al. has shown the anti-pruritic effect of 5% doxepin in AD patients.[77] In addition, topical mast cell stabilizers, such as sodium cromoglycate, have also shown some potential.[78]

Although the evidence is still rudimentary, but topical N-palmitoylethanolamine, capsaicin, doxepin and sodium cromoglycate may be effective as adjuvant antipruritic therapies in AE.[14] Further RCT are required to conclusively recommend routine use in AD.

UV Therapy

UV irradiation relieves pruritus in AD and NB-UVB seems to be more effective than UVA and UVA1.[14]

Oral Antihistamines

Traditionally, oral antihistamines have been used in the management of pruritus in patients with AD, but there is insufficient evidence to recommend the general use of antihistamines as part of the treatment of AD.[53]

A systematic review[74] showed that nonsedating histamines are ineffectual in AD management. Moreover, the use of both sedating and nonsedating medications has revealed mixed results and favors no benefit, with many patients reporting as much improvement with placebo.[79] Nevertheless, short-term, intermittent use of sedating antihistamines may be beneficial in the setting of sleep loss secondary to itch, but should not be substituted for management of AD with topical therapies.[53]

Other Systemic Antipruritic Agents

Although systemic immunosuppressive agents, such as glucocorticosteroids or cyclosporine does appears to partly abolish pruritus, but no specific studies on an anti-itch effect in AD were published.[14]

Similarly, opioid-receptor antagonists naltrexone[80] and nalmefene[81] may reduce AD itch, but there is insufficient data to recommend routine use of these substances in AD.[14]

NONPHARMACOLOGIC INTERVENTIONS

Dietary Interventions and Supplements

The absolute benefit from dietary restriction in AD is yet to be proven as studies fail to provide conclusive evidence.[82] Although, some evidence shows that avoidance of foods to which there is a known sensitivity may reduce the severity and extent of AD, but causality is difficult to establish when this is tested and there is a frequent misattribution of AD flares to food-related issues. Food allergies may coexist and represent important triggers in a small subset of individuals with AD but the true frequency of food allergies causing an isolated flare of disease is probably low.[83] Moreover, when the allergen is food, excessive restriction can lead to nutrition deficiency.

There may be some benefit to an egg-free diet in infants with suspected egg allergy who also have positive specific IgE to eggs, but other exclusion diets (e.g, milk-free, elemental, few-foods diets) were not found to be efficacious in unselected AD populations.[84] Suspicious triggers should be recorded in a diary and food diary and diagnostic elimination should be tried for 4–6 weeks following a consistent correlation. Symptomatic improvement warrants an oral food challenge for confirmation.[85,86]

Patients with AD might benefit from supplementation with vitamin D, particularly if they have a documented low level or low vitamin D intake.[87] However, topical vitamin D preparations are to be avoided because they might worsen eczematous dermatitis through both allergic and irritant mechanisms.[88]

In addition, most studies suggest no therapeutic efficacy of essential fatty acids (evening primrose oil, borage oil), pyridoxine, vitamin E, multivitamins, and zinc supplementation as results from studies failed to achieve reduction in extent and severity of AD.[26,89,90,91]

Probiotics are defined as live organisms that can confer beneficial effects on the health of the host. They down-regulate production of Th2 cytokines (*e.g.*, IL-4, IL-13) and up-regulate production of either Th1 cytokines (*e.g.*, IL-12, IFN-γ) or regulatory T cells (*e.g.*, IL-10, TGF-β) in vitro,[92] but these findings have not been replicated in vivo.[93] Studies examining the use of probiotics for the prevention and treatment of atopic disease have revealed conflicting results.[93] In the absence of independent conformation, none of the latest guidelines on AD treatment advocate its use in AD.[5,26,48,86] Nonetheless, probiotics continue to be viewed as an effective strategy for the management of this disease.

Psychodermatological Aspects and Psychological Interventions

Psychological factors are important in the treatment of chronic dermatological conditions like AD as there is no cure and patients often experience a lifelong struggle with the condition.[94] Though not caused by stress, AD itself causes stress and also appears to be precipitated or exacerbated by it.[95] This interplay of emotional factors which may determine the natural course of the disease pushes AD under the domain of psychophysiological disorder.[95]

An understanding of a patient's mental burden of anxiety, difficulties in dealing with anger, depressive symptoms associated with greater severity of pruritus and excitability is essential for successful psychodermatological treatment.[96] This can be achieved by a good doctor-patient relationship as treatment alone may not be enough for long-term management and high-quality consultations are necessary for adherence to treatment during the course of chronicity and flare-up of the disease.[97] The best approach is to observe both the skin and the psyche during the consultation, assessing the patient's mental status while maintaining a level of empathy or even compassion toward the patient. It is important to focus on the impact of the disease on QoL, and talking about the influence of stress and unresolved traumatic experiences is essential.[94]

Psychological interventions that have been studied include autogenic training, biofeedback, brief dynamic psychotherapy, cognitive behavioral therapy, habit reversal behavioral therapy, and a stress management program.[86,98] Although the quality of evidence for these interventions is poor, a more robust evaluation may lead to reliable benefits.[99] In the absence of any studies from India, it is difficult to make any recommendation for our setting as these are specialist interventions.

Environmental Modifications

Although suggested as potential triggers for the development, severity and exacerbation of atopic eczema, level of evidence for manipulation of environmental factors remains poor.[26] The clinical benefit from reduction of house-dust-mite allergen or pet exposure remains unclear[48] as studies failed to demonstrate improvement in AD severity following cleaning measures.[86,100,101]

Use of cotton and avoidance of wool has been recommended in the past. Contrary to this belief, cotton clothing did not confer any benefits when compared to other fabrics constructed with smooth fibers.[48] However, limited evidence suggests that silver-coated textiles[102] due to a possible antibacterial effect or silk with or without added antimicrobial agent[103,104] can reduce AD symptoms.

Although good-quality trials are lacking, nevertheless whenever any irritant effect is suspected, avoidance of biological washing powders, fabric conditioners and fragrance products, such as soaps and shower gels should be advised.[26,86]

Educational Interventions

In AD, understanding the disease is as important as medical care, because many factors contribute to the pathogenesis of AD.[105] Knowledge of AD of both patients and their parents, and compliance with AD management practices are important to improve clinical outcomes.[105]

A recent Cochrane review[99] recognizes two main service delivery models for education—nurse-led and multidisciplinary therapeutic patient and/or parent education. In some countries, such as the UK, nurse-led clinics provide an opportunity for focused intervention; however the evidence that parental education delivered by nurses who are caring for children with atopic eczema may improve the clinical severity of the atopic eczema is limited. Evidence from German multicenter study[106] of multidisciplinary intervention using an eczema school curriculum indicates that children and their parental carers may benefit from structured education, albeit using a complex intervention.

The American Academy of Dermatology also recommends educational programs (i.e. training programs and "eczema schools"), video interventions, eczema workshops and nurse-led programs as an adjunct to the conventional therapy of AD (Fig. 5.3).[86,107-113]

COMPLEMENTARY AND ALTERNATIVE MEDICINE[114,115]

World over patients with chronic skin ailments do resort to alternative medicines which are not part of conventional or allopathic or traditional mainstream medicine, the so called standard care practices. People resort to these remedies because of various reasons, such as the nonallopathic physicians spending more time with their patients, the nonallopathic drugs are expected to have less side effects, the cost involved or the high amount of adverse effects and sometimes ineffectiveness

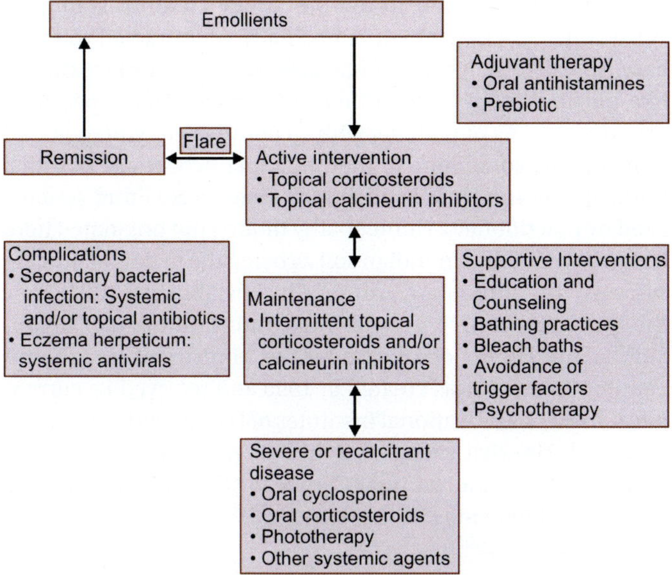

Fig. 5.3: Treatment algorithm for atopic dermatitis

of the drugs used by allopaths. Various names are given to these remedies, such as alternate medicines, complimentary medicines and integrative medicine. By definition alternative medicines are therapies which are used in "diagnosis, treatment or prevention of diseases or ill-health and maintenance of health by complementing mainstream or so called allopathic medicine, by contributing to a common goal or by integrating or all by itself and, by satisfying a demand not met by the conventional medicine alone. There are several methods, such as biologically- or physically-based practices, whole medical systems, mind and body medicines, manipulative and such others as music, relaxation, etc.

Atopic dermatitis being a chronic relapsing disease where conventional treatment with allopathy or scientific medicine has its own limitations and adverse reactions, patients tend to take these alternate medicines before, during and even afterwards.

World over every region has their own medical systems, such as Chinese, Tibetan, Japanese, native American, etc. Our own Indian system of Ayurveda and yoga systems are used frequently by many patients. Various other forms are— Chinese, acupuncture and acupressure, Ayurveda and yoga, unani, herbal medicines, chiropractice, aroma therapy, massages, music, dietary manipulation, vitamins, naturopathy and minerals, reflexology, etc. many of these modalities give cure rates in anecdotal patients but lack in clear evidence to support. Also some of them may have adverse effects. Still the modalities are popular in masses. Many citations state that various percentage of people normally get attracted to these easy, so called natural and harmless modalities of treatment like music therapy, aroma therapy, etc. In editors, personal experience, 60% of patients with AD have used Ayurveda and homeopathy some time in their therapeutic travails. In India, homeopathy and Unani and Siddha systems are other systems used by practitioners. Homeopathy though not originated here has strong foothold in Indian soil as being the major healthcare systems. The Indian government has established AYUSH or the Department of Ayurveda, Yoga and Naturopathy, Unani, Siddha and Homoeopathy under the Ministry of Health and Family Welfare; It was created in 1995 and received its current name in 2003. The National Institutes of Health (NIH) in United States of America recognizes use of Alternative Medicine and has initiated a National Center for Complementary and Alternative Medicine (NCCAM) in 1998.

AYURVEDA

Ayurveda meaning science of life works on principle that body is made up of three doshas and depending on imbalance of these and basic body type of patient, remedy is offered to balance the doshas. According to "Charak Samhita" that is pharmacopoeia of Ayurveda, eczemas can come in group of vicharchikas and medicines can be offered to cure it. Herbs like "aloe vera" can be soothing and help in reducing itch and improve barrier function.

HOMEOPATHY[116]

Homeopathy was initiated by Samuel Hahnemann (1755–1843), a German physician who later moved to Paris. The word "homeopathy" is derived from the Greek words *Homoios* ("similar") and *pathos* ("feeling or suffering"). The method is based on the law of similars and on the law of infinitesimals.

The first law denotes the assumption that symptoms in diseased individual can be cured by a drug which is able to induce the same symptoms in a healthy individual. The second law defines the rule that the appropriate drug has to be given in high dilutions, and that the higher the dilution, the greater the effect (so-called potentiation). Modern physics and chemistry have shown that some of the dilutions used in homeopathy are so high that virtually no single molecule of the original substance remains in the preparation. For treating physicians however, the "essence" of the original substance is considered to remain in the water, hypothesis of so called "retention of memory" has been postulated.

Because atopic eczema does spontaneously wax and wane, many alternative healers claim to the patient or their parents that the drug has caused an improvement. For example, a patient whose itching has improved after few years is because of medicines. It is important to realize that homeopathy is a concept based on belief that cannot be falsified by any scientific research. It is based on some irrational belief and it is supposed to give holistic approach rather than diagnostic therapy.

ACUPUNCTURE

Acupuncture—needle acupuncture is traditional Chinese way of healing. It is practiced since 300 years. It was used in pain and since itch works on same pathways, it also might help in AD itch. The needles are inserted in specific points at and around nerves and plexus and kept for half an hour, treatment repeated weekly or biweekly. The process may act by interfering nerve impulses and/or releasing cytokines.

ADVERSE EFFECTS

Adverse Effects of CAM

Direct side effects from the constituents of a homeopathic drug, may be rare because of the extremely-high dilutions used.

There may also be indirect side effects due to withdrawal of an effective treatment. As direct side effects, chromate dermatitis due to homeopathic preparations and baboon syndrome with pronounced flexural erythema triggered by mercury have been reported.

CONCLUSION

The alternative medicine is here to stay. It offers romanticism, more natural than artificial, chemical and technical. We should respect patients freedom to choose but all the same protect them from further financial burden, worsening, sufferings and fallacies of the practitioners themselves, simultaneously emphasizing the advantages and disadvantages of so called main theme medicines. Very often it is a search for emotional help, better coping with the disease, or the impression of more active participation in the healing process. The patients who were using alternate medicines were seen to have severe disease, poor QOL, lower socio-economic group and less educated (at personal observation).

REFERENCES

1. McKenna SP, Doward LC. Quality of life of children with atopic dermatitis and their families. Curr Opin Allergy Clin Immunol. 2008;8:228-31.
2. Cork MJ, Britton J, Butler L, Young S, Murphy R, Keohane SG. Comparison of parent knowledge, therapy utilization and severity of atopic eczema before and after explanation and demonstration of topical therapies by a specialist dermatology nurse. Br J Dermatol. 2003;149:582-9.
3. Staab D, Diepgen TL, Fartasch M, et al. Age related, structured educational programmes for the management of atopic dermatitis in children and adolescents: multicentre, randomised controlled trial. BMJ. 2006;332:933-8.
4. Schneider L, Tilles S, Lio P, et al. Atopic dermatitis: a practice parameter update 2012. J Allergy Clin Immunol. 2013;131:295-9.
5. Eichenfield LF, Tom WL, Berger TG, et al. Guidelines of care for the management of atopic dermatitis. J Am Acad Dermatol. 2014;71:116-32.
6. Varothai S, Nitayavardhana S, Kulthanan K. Moisturizers for patients with atopic dermatitis. Asian Pac J Allergy Immunol. 2013;31:91-8.
7. Breternitz M, Kowatzki D, Langenauer M, Elsner P, Fluhr JW. Placebo-controlled, double-blind, randomized, prospective study of a glycerol-based emollient on eczematous skin in atopic dermatitis: biophysical and clinical evaluation. Skin Pharmacol Physiol. 2008;21:39-45.
8. Peris K, Valeri P, Altobelli E, Fargnoli MC, Carrozzo AM, Chimenti S. Efficacy evaluation of an oil-in-water emulsion (Dermoflan) in atopic dermatitis. Acta Derm Venereol. 2002;82:465-6.
9. Grimalt R, Mengeaud V, Cambazard F; Study Investigators' Group. The steroid-sparing effect of an emollient therapy in infants with atopic dermatitis: a randomized controlled study. Dermatology. 2007;214:61-7.
10. Msika P, De Belilovsky C, Piccardi N, Chebassier N, Baudouin C, Chadoutaud B. New emollient with topical corticosteroid-sparing effect in treatment of childhood atopic dermatitis: SCORAD and quality of life improvement. Pediatr Dermatol. 2008;25:606-12.
11. Draelos ZD. An evaluation of prescription device moisturizers. J Cosmet Dermatol. 2009;8:40-3.
12. Wollenberg A, Wetzel S, Burgdorf WH, et al. Viral infections in atopic dermatitis: pathogenic aspects and clinical management. J Allergy Clin Immunol. 2003;112:667-74.

13. Hon KL, Ching GK, Leung TF, Choi CY, Lee KK, Ng PC. Estimating emollient usage in patients with eczema. Clin Exp Dermatol. 2010;35:22-6.
14. Ring J, Alomar A, Bieber T, et al. Guidelines for treatment of atopic eczema (atopic dermatitis) part I. J Eur Acad Dermatol Venereol. 2012;26:1045-60.
15. Gutman AB, Kligman AM, Sciacca J, James WD. Soak and smear: a standard technique revisited. Arch Dermatol. 2005;141:1556-9.
16. Chiang C, Eichenfield LF. Quantitative assessment of combination bathing and moisturizing regimens on skin hydration in atopic dermatitis. Pediatr Dermatol. 2009;26:273-8.
17. Simpson E, Trookman NS, Rizer RL, et al. Safety and tolerability of a body wash and moisturizer when applied to infants and toddlers with a history of atopic dermatitis: results from an open-label study. Pediatr Dermatol. 2012;29:590-7.
18. Ananthapadmanabhan KP, Moore DJ, Subramanyan K, Misra M, Meyer F. Cleansing without compromise: the impact of cleansers on the skin barrier and the technology of mild cleansing. Dermatol Ther. 2004;17(Suppl 1):16-25.
19. White MI, Jenkinson DM, Lloyd DH. The effect of washing on the thickness of the stratum corneum in normal and atopic individuals. Br J Dermatol. 1987;116:525-30.
20. Solodkin G, Chaudhari U, Subramanyan K, Johnson AW, Yan X, Gottlieb A. Benefits of mild cleansing: synthetic surfactant based (syndet) bars for patients with atopic dermatitis. Cutis. 2006;77:317-24.
21. Cheong WK. Gentle cleansing and moisturizing for patients with atopic dermatitis and sensitive skin. Am J Clin Dermatol. 2009;10(Suppl 1):13-7.
22. Hon KL, Leung TF, Wong Y, So HK, Li AM, Fok TF. A survey of bathing and showering practices in children with atopic eczema. Clin Exp Dermatol. 2005;30(4):351-4.
23. Devillers AC, Oranje AP. Efficacy and safety of 'wet-wrap' dressings as an intervention treatment in children with severe and/or refractory atopic dermatitis: a critical review of the literature. Br J Dermatol. 2006;154:579-85.
24. Dabade TS, Davis DM, Wetter DA, et al. Wet dressing therapy in conjunction with topical corticosteroids is effective for rapid control of severe pediatric atopic dermatitis: experience with 218 patients over 30 years at Mayo Clinic. J Am Acad Dermatol. 2012;67:100-6.
25. Leung DYM, Boguniewicz M, Howell MD, Nomura I, Hamid QA. New insights into atopic dermatitis. J Clin Invest. 2004;113:651-7.
26. Scottish Intercollegiate Guidelines Network (SIGN). Management of atopic eczema in primary care. Edinburgh: SIGN; 2011. (SIGN publication no. 125). [March 2011]. Available from URL: http://www.sign.ac.uk.

27. National Collaborating Centre for Women's and Children's Health (UK). Atopic Eczema in Children: Management of Atopic Eczema in Children from Birth up to the Age of 12 Years. London: RCOG Press; 2007 Dec. (NICE Clinical Guidelines, No. 57.) Available from: http://www.ncbi.nlm.nih.gov/books/NBK49365/

28. Thomas KS, Armstrong S, Avery A, et al. Randomized controlled trial of short bursts of a potent topical corticosteroid versus prolonged use of a mild preparation for children with mild or moderate atopic eczema. BMJ. 2002;324:768.

29. Hebert AA. Desonide foam 0.05%: safety in children as young as 3 months. J Am Acad Dermatol. 2008;59:334-40.

30. Williams HC. Established corticosteroid creams should be applied only once daily in patients with atopic eczema. BMJ. 2007;334:1272.

31. Callen, J, Chamlin S, Eichenfield LF, et al. A systematic review of the safety of topical therapies for atopic dermatitis. Br J Dermatol. 2007;156:203-21.

32. Schmitt J, von Kobyletzki L, Svensson A, Apfelbacher C. Efficacy and tolerability of proactive treatment with topical corticosteroids and calcineurin inhibitors for atopic eczema: systematic review and meta-analysis of randomized controlled trials. Br J Dermatol. 2011;164:415-28.

33. Ellison JA, Patel L, Ray DW, David TJ, Clayton PE. Hypothalamic-pituitary-adrenal function and glucocorticoid sensitivity in atopic dermatitis. Pediatrics. 2000;105:794-9.

34. Charman CR, Morris, AD, Williams HC. Topical corticosteroid phobia in patients with atopic eczema. Br J Dermatol. 2000;142:931-6.

35. Cork MJ, Britton J, Butler L, Young S, Murphy R, Keohane SG. Comparison of parent knowledge, therapy utilization and severity of atopic eczema before and after explanation and demonstration of topical therapies by a specialist dermatology nurse. Br J Dermatol. 2003;149:582-9.

36. Ashcroft DM, Dimmock P, Garside R, Stein K, Williams HC. Efficacy and tolerability of topical pimecrolimus and tacrolimus in the treatment of atopic dermatitis: meta-analysis of randomised controlled trials. BMJ. 2005;330:516.

37. Luger T, Van Leent EJ, Graeber M, et al. SDZ ASM 981: an emerging safe and effective treatment for atopic dermatitis. Br J Dermatol. 2001;144:788-94.

38. Abramovits W, Fleischer AB Jr, Jaracz E, Breneman D. Adult patients with moderate atopic dermatitis: tacrolimus ointment versus pimecrolimus cream. J Drugs Dermatol. 2008;7:1153-8.

39. Fleischer AB Jr, Abramovits W, Breneman D, Jaracz E. Tacrolimus ointment is more effective than pimecrolimus cream in adult patients with moderate to very severe atopic dermatitis. J Dermatology Treat. 2007;18:151-7.

40. Kapp A, Papp K, Bingham A, et al. Long-term management of atopic dermatitis in infants with topical pimecrolimus, a nonsteroid anti-inflammatory drug. J Allergy Clin Immunol. 2002;110:277-84.
41. Murrell DF, Calvieri S, Ortonne JP, et al. A randomized controlled trial of pimecrolimus cream 1% in adolescents and adults with head and neck atopic dermatitis and intolerant of, or dependent on, topical corticosteroids. Br J Dermatol. 2007;157:954-9.
42. El-Batawy MM, Bosseila MA, Mashaly HM, Hafez VS. Topical calcineurin inhibitors in atopic dermatitis: a systematic review and meta-analysis. J Dermatol Sci. 2009;54:76-87.
43. Reitamo S, Harper J, Bos JD, et al. 0.03% Tacrolimus ointment applied once or twice daily is more efficacious than 1% hydrocortisone acetate in children with moderate to severe atopic dermatitis: results of a randomized double-blind controlled trial. Br J Dermatol. 2004;150:554-62.
44. Ruer-Mulard M, Aberer W, Gunstone A, et al. Twice-daily versus once-daily applications of pimecrolimus cream 1% for the prevention of disease relapse in pediatric patients with atopic dermatitis. Pediatr Dermatol. 2009;26:551-8.
45. Breneman D, Fleischer AB Jr, Abramovits W, et al. Intermittent therapy for flare prevention and long-term disease control in stabilized atopic dermatitis: a randomized comparison of 3-times-weekly applications of tacrolimus ointment versus vehicle. J Am Acad Dermatol. 2008;58:990-9.
46. Paller AS, Eichenfield LF, Kirsner RS, Shull T, Jaracz E, Simpson EL. Three times weekly tacrolimus ointment reduces relapse in stabilized atopic dermatitis: a new paradigm for use. Pediatrics. 2008;122:e1210-8.
47. Tennis P, Gelfand JM, Rothman KJ. Evaluation of cancer risk related to atopic dermatitis and use of topical calcineurin inhibitors. Br J Dermatol. 2011;165:465-73.
48. Hoare C, Li Wan Po A, Williams H. Systematic review of treatments for atopic eczema. Health Technol Assess. 2000;4:1-191.
49. Slutsky JB, Clark RA, Remedios AA, Klein PA. An evidence-based review of the efficacy of coal tar preparations in the treatment of psoriasis and atopic dermatitis. J Drugs Dermatol. 2010;9:1258-64.
50. Niordson AM, Stahl D. Treatment of psoriasis with Clinitar Cream. A controlled clinical trial. Br J Clin Pract. 1985;39:67-8, 72.
51. Roelofzen JH, Aben KK, Oldenhof UT, et al. No increased risk of cancer after coal tar treatment in patients with psoriasis or eczema. J Invest Dermatol. 2010;130:953-61.
52. Meduri NB, Vandergriff T, Rasmussen H, Jacobe H. Phototherapy in the management of atopic dermatitis: a systematic review. Photodermatol Photoimmunol Photomed. 2007;23:106-12.

53. Sidbury R, Davis DM, Cohen DE, Cordoro KM, Berger TG, Bergman JN. Guidelines of care for the management of atopic dermatitis: section 3. Management and treatment with phototherapy and systemic agents. J Am Acad Dermatol. 2014;71:327-49.

54. Astellas. Medication guide (tacrolimus). Available from: URL:http://www.protopic.com/pdf/protopic_med_guide.pdf. Accessed October 9, 2014.

55. Medicis. Prescribing information (pimecrolimus). Available from: URL:http://elidel-us.com/files/Elidel_PI.pdf. Accessed October 9, 2014.

56. Prinz B, Michelsen S, Pfeiffer C, Plewig G. Long-term application of extracorporeal photochemotherapy in severe atopic dermatitis. J Am Acad Dermatol. 1999;40:577-82.

57. Menter A, Korman NJ, Elmets CA, et al. Guidelines of care for the management of psoriasis and psoriatic arthritis, section 5: guidelines of care for the treatment of psoriasis with phototherapy and photochemotherapy. J Am Acad Dermatol. 2010;62:114-35.

58. van Joost T, Heule F, Korstanje M, van den Broek MJ, Stenveld HJ, van Vloten WA. Cyclosporin in atopic dermatitis: a multicenter placebo-controlled study. Br J Dermatol. 1994;130:634-40.

59. Sowden JM, Berth-Jones J, Ross JS, et al. Double-blind, controlled, crossover study of cyclosporin in adults with severe refractory atopic dermatitis. Lancet. 1991;338:137-40.

60. Berth-Jones J, Finlay AY, Zaki I, et al. Cyclosporine in severe childhood atopic dermatitis: a multicenter study. J Am Acad Dermatol. 1996;34:1016-21.

61. Akdis CA, Akdis M, Bieber T, et al. Diagnosis and treatment of atopic dermatitis in children and adults: European Academy of Allergology and Clinical Immunology/American Academy of Allergy, Asthma and Immunology/PRACTALL Consensus Report. J Allergy Clin Immunol. 2006;118:152-69.

62. Schram ME, Roekevisch E, Leeflang MM, Bos JD, Schmitt J, Spuls PI. A randomized trial of methotrexate versus azathioprine for severe atopic eczema. J Allergy Clin Immunol. 2011;128:353-9.

63. Guttman-Yassky E, Dhingra N, Leung DY. New era of biologic therapeutics in atopic dermatitis. Expert Opin Biol Ther. 2013;13:549-61.

64. Denby KS, Beck LA. Update on systemic therapies for atopic dermatitis. Curr Opin Allergy Clin Immunol. 2012;12: 421-6.

65. Ong PY, Boguniewicz M. Investigational and unproven therapies in atopic dermatitis. Immunol Allergy Clin North Am. 2010;30:425-39.

66. Hanifin JM, Schneider LC, Leung DY, et al. Recombinant interferon gamma therapy for atopic dermatitis. J Am Acad Dermatol. 1993;28(2 Pt 1):189-97.

67. Jang IG, Yang JK, Lee HJ, et al. Clinical improvement and immunohistochemical findings in severe atopic dermatitis treated with interferon gamma. J Am Acad Dermatol. 2000;42:1033-40.

68. Ring J, Alomar A, Bieber T, et al. Guidelines for treatment of atopic eczema (atopic dermatitis) Part II. J Eur Acad Dermatol Venereol. 2012;26:1176-93.

69. Takei S, Arora YK, Walker SM. Intravenous immunoglobulin contains specific antibodies inhibitory to activation of T cells by staphylococcal toxin superantigens. J Clin Invest. 1993;91:602-7.

70. Jolles S. A review of high-dose intravenous immunoglobulin treatment for atopic dermatits. Clin Exp Dermatol. 2002;27:3-7.

71. Boguniewicz M, Sampson H, Leung SB, Harbeck R, Leung DY. Effects of cefuroxime axetil on *Staphylococcus aureus* colonization and superantigen production in atopic dermatitis. J Allergy Clin Immunol. 2001;108:651-2.

72. Bath-Hextall FJ, Birnie AJ, Ravenscroft JC, Williams HC. Interventions to reduce *Staphylococcus aureus* in the management of atopic eczema: an updated Cochrane review. Br J Dermatol. 2010;163:12-26.

73. Sher LG, Chang J, Patel IB, Balkrishnan R, Fleischer AB Jr. Relieving the pruritus of atopic dermatitis: a meta-analysis. Acta Derm Venereol. 2012;92:455-61.

74. Klein PA, Clark RA. An evidence-based review of the efficacy of antihistamines in relieving pruritus in atopic dermatitis. Arch Dermatol. 1999;135:1522-5.

75. Eberlein B, Eicke C, Reinhardt HW, Ring J. Adjuvant treatment of atopic eczema: assessment of an emollient containing N-palmitoylethanolamine (ATOPA study). J Eur Acad Dermatol Venereol. 2008;22:73-82.

76. Weisshaar E, Heyer G, Forster C. Effect of topical capsaicin on the cutaneous reactions and itching to histamine in atopic eczema patients compared to healthy skin. Arch Dermatol Res. 1998;290:306.

77. Drake LA, Fallon JD, Sober A. Relief of pruritus in patients with atopic dermatitis after treatment with topical doxepin cream. The Doxepin Study Group. J Am Acad Dermatol. 1994;31:613-6.

78. Stainer R, Matthews S, Arshad SH, et al. Efficacy and acceptability of a new topical skin lotion of sodium cromoglicate (Altoderm) in atopic dermatitis in children aged 2–12 years: a double-blind, randomized, placebo-controlled trial. Br J Dermatol. 2005;152:334-41.

79. Epstein E, Pinski JB. A blind study. Arch Dermatol. 1964;89:548-9.

80. Malekzad F, Arbabi M, Mohtasham N, et al. Efficacy of oral naltrexone on pruritus in atopic eczema: a double-blind,

placebo-controlled study. J Eur Acad Dermatol Venereol. 2009;23:948-50.

81. Monroe EW. Efficacy and safety of nalmefene in patients with severe pruritus caused by chronic urticaria and atopic dermatitis. J Am Acad Dermatol. 1989;21:135-6.

82. Sloper KS, Wadsworth J, Brostoff J. Children with atopic eczema I: Clinical response to food elimination and subsequent double-blind food challenge. Q J Med. 1991;80: 677-93.

83. Rowlands D, Tofte SJ, Hanifin JM. Does food allergy cause atopic dermatitis? Food challenge testing to dissociate eczematous from immediate reactions. Dermatol Ther. 2006;19:97-103.

84. Bath-Hextall F, Delamere FM, Williams HC. Dietary exclusions for established atopic eczema. Cochrane Database Syst Rev. 2008;1:CD005203.

85. Werfel T, Ballmer-Weber B, Eigenmann PA, et al. Eczematous reactions to food in atopic eczema: position paper of the EAACI and GA2LEN. Allergy. 2007;62:723-8.

86. Sidbury R, Tom WL, Bergman JN, Cooper KD, Silverman RA, Berger TG. Guidelines of care for the management of atopic dermatitis: Section 4. Prevention of disease flares and use of adjunctive therapies and approaches. J Am Acad Dermatol. 2014;71:1218-33.

87. Sidbury R, Sullivan AF, Thadhani RI, Camargo CA. Randomized controlled trial of vitamin D supplementation for winter-related atopic dermatitis in Boston: a pilot study. Br J Dermatol. 2009;159:245-7.

88. Feily A, Namazi MR. Vitamin A + D ointment is not an appropriate emollient for atopic dermatitis. Dermatitis. 2010;21:174-5.

89. Berth-Jones J, Graham-Brown RA. Placebo-controlled trial of essential fatty acid supplementation in atopic dermatitis. Lancet. 1993;341:1557-60.

90. Mabin DC, Hollis S, Lockwood J, et al. Pyridoxine in atopic dermatitis. Br J Dermatol. 1995;133:764-7.

91. Ewing CI, Gibbs AC, Ashcroft C, et al. Failure of oral zinc supplementation in atopic eczema. Eur J Clin Nutr. 1991;45:507-10.

92. van der Aa LB, Heymans HS, van Aalderen WM, Sprikkelman AB. Probiotics and prebiotics in atopic dermatitis: review of the theoretical background and clinical evidence. Pediatr Allergy Immunol. 2010;21:e355-67.

93. Yang HJ, Min TK, Lee HW, Pyun BY. Efficacy of Probiotic Therapy on Atopic Dermatitis in Children: A Randomized, Double-blind, Placebo-controlled Trial. Allergy Asthma Immunol Res. 2014;6:208-15.

94. Senra MS, Wollenberg A. Psychodermatological aspects of atopic dermatitis. Br J Dermatology. 2014;170 (Suppl s1): 38-43.

95. Morren MA, Przybilla B, Bamelis M, et al. Atopic dermatitis: triggering factors. J Am Acad Dermatol. 1994;31:467-73.
96. Jafferany M. Psychodermatology: a guide to understanding common psychocutaneous disorders. Prim Care Companion J Clin Psychiatry. 2007;9:203-13.
97. Poot F. Doctor-patient relations in dermatology: obligations and rights for a mutual satisfaction. J Eur Acad Dermatol Venereol. 2009;23:1233-9.
98. Chida Y, Steptoe A, Hirakawa N, Sudo N, Kubo C. The effects of psychological intervention on atopic dermatitis: A systematic review and meta-analysis. Int Arch Allergy Immunol. 2007;144:1-9.
99. Ersser SJ, Cowdell F, Latter S, et al. Psychological and educational interventions for atopic eczema in children. Cochrane Database of Systematic Reviews. 2014;1:CD004054.
100. Gutgesell C, Heise S, Seubert S, et al. Double-blind placebo-controlled house dust mite control measures in adult patients with atopic dermatitis. Br J Dermatol. 2001;145:70-4.
101. Friedmann PS, Tan BB. Mite elimination—clinical effect on eczema. Allergy. 1998;53:97-100.
102. Gauger A, Fischer S, Mempel M, et al. Efficacy and functionality of silver-coated textiles in patients with atopic eczema. J Eur Acad Dermatol Venereol. 2006;20:534-41.
103. Ricci G, Patrizi A, Bendandi B, Menna G, Varotti E, Masi M. Clinical effectiveness of a silk fabric in the treatment of atopic dermatitis. Br J Dermatol. 2004;150:127-31.
104. Senti G, Steinmann LS, Fischer B, et al. Antimicrobial silk clothing in the treatment of atopic dermatitis proves comparable to topical corticosteroid treatment. Dermatology. 2006;213:228-33.
105. Shin JY, Kim do W, Park CW, Seo SJ, Park YL, Lee JR. An educational program that contributes to improved patient and parental understanding of atopic dermatitis. Ann Dermatol. 2014;26:66-72.
106. Kupfer J, Gieler U, Diepgen TL, Fartasch M, Lob-Corzilius T, Ring J, et al. Structured education program improves the coping with atopic dermatitis in children and their parents—a multicenter, randomized controlled trial. J Psychosom Res. 2010;68:353-8.
107. Cole WC, Roth HL, Sachs LB. Group psychotherapy as an aid in the medical treatment of eczema. J Am Acad Dermatol. 1988;18:286-91.
108. Schmitt J, Schmitt N, Meurer M. Cyclosporin in the treatment of patients with atopic eczema—a systematic review and meta-analysis. J Eur Acad Dermatol Venereol. 2007;21:606-19.
109. Guttman-Yassky E, Dhingra N, Leung DY. New Era of Biological Therapeutics in Atopic Dermatitis. Expert Opin Biol Ther. 2013;13:549-61.

110. Saeki H, Furue M, Furukawa F, et al. Guidelines for management of atopic dermatitis. J Dermatol. 2009;36:563-77.

111. Cork MJ, Britton J, Butler L, Young S, Murphy R, Keohane SG. Comparison of parent knowledge, therapy utilization and severity of atopic eczema before and after explanation and demonstration of topical therapies by a specialist dermatology nurse. Br J Dermatol. 2003;149:582-9.

112. Ben-Gashir MA, Seed PT, Hay RJ. Quality of life and disease severity are correlated in children with atopic dermatitis. Br J Dermatol. 2004;150:284-90.

113. Armstrong AW, Kim RH, Idriss NZ, Larsen LN, Lio PA. Online video improves clinical outcomes in adults with atopic dermatitis: a randomized controlled trial. J Am Acad Dermatol. 2011;64:502-7.

114 Artik S, Ruzicka T. Complementary therapy for atopic eczema and other allergic skin diseases. Dermatol Ther. 2003;16:150-163.

115. Bielory L. Complementory medicine for the allergist. Allergy Asthma Proc. 2001;22(1):33-7.

116. Burgdorf WHC, Happle R. What every dermatologist should know about homeopathy. Arch Dermatol. 1996;132:955-8.

Index

Page numbers followed by *f* refer to figure and *t* refer to table.